Integrative Group Therapy for Psychosis

Stemming from a series of outcome and process studies, this book presents an evidence-based, integrative group therapy treatment model that includes elements from psychodynamic, interpersonal, psychoeducational, and cognitive-behavioral approaches to address the needs of people suffering from psychosis.

Designed to help patients deal with delusions, hallucinations, disorganized thinking, interpersonal problems, mood changes, and the stigma of having a serious mental illness, the book chronicles the evolution of the integrative approach from research in inpatient and outpatient settings to theoretical and clinical issues that were derived from the empirical studies. Chapters also include information and vignettes to assist the reader in conducting therapy groups for patients suffering from psychosis, including schizophrenia spectrum and bipolar disorders.

Shown to be a safe and supportive adjunct to medications that is useful in both inpatient and outpatient settings, readers will find value in this unique, empirically driven model for groups that are long-term, short-term, and time-limited.

Nick Kanas, MD, is Professor Emeritus (Psychiatry) at the University of California, San Francisco (UCSF). He has conducted clinical and research work on group therapy at the San Francisco Veterans Hospital, UCSF, and other national and international settings. He has been leading therapy groups for psychotic patients since 1975, and his first book on the subject was *Group Therapy for Schizophrenic Patients.*

"In this excellent and well written text, Dr. Kanas thoughtfully illustrates the implementation of group therapy for individuals with psychotic disorders. Advancing well beyond the limitations of traditional, theoretical singularity, Kanas' integrative approach brings to life a model of group therapy that addresses the human experience that lies beneath our patients' manifest symptomatology. This book describes in clear and useful fashion how group therapy improves patients' interpersonal engagement and self-efficacy, in the context of chronic and recurrent major mental illnesses."

Molyn Leszcz, MD, FRCPC, CGP, DFAGPA, Professor of Psychiatry, University of Toronto; President, American Group Psychotherapy Association

"A masterful piece of clinical scholarship representing over four decades of dedicated study of group psychological treatments for psychotic level pathologies. In a creative and comprehensive manner, filled with illuminating clinical vignettes, Dr. Kanas brings together the best of what too often are isolated schools of psychotherapy—psychodynamic, interpersonal, psychoeducational, and cognitive behavioral. This is a compelling and authoritative work, backed by keen clinical observation and empirical evidence, that should serve as a mainstay for all who face the challenges of psychological work in groups with this difficult clinical population."

Les R. Greene, PhD, Past President, American Group Psychotherapy Association; Clinical Faculty, Yale University School of Medicine; Co-editor, *Core Principles of Group Psychotherapy: An Integrated Theory, Research, and Practice Training Manual (2019)*

"Dr. Kanas's *Integrative Group Therapy for Psychosis: An Evidence-Based Approach is a* **must read** for clinicians. The historical chapter is comprehensive, succinct, and provides a vital understanding of the types of group treatment offered to people with psychotic conditions over the past several decades. I loved the clinical and personal richness added by the excerpts from Robert Francis who suffers from chronic schizophrenia throughout the book! The integrative model presented incorporates the rigor of science and the wisdom of an experienced clinician."

Gary M. Burlingame, PhD, CGP, APA, Fellow and DFAGPA; President-elect, AGPA; Professor and Chair of Psychology, Brigham Young University

"Finally, there is a book addressing the powerful impact that group therapy provides a severely neglected population, those people struggling with psychotic disorders. Dr. Kanas does an excellent job reviewing the literature, describing the integration of dynamic, cognitive-behavioral, and interpersonal theories, and summarizing the research and work he has been done (sic) over the course of his life. Not only does Dr. Kanas educate us about the strong evidence supporting this group treatment, but he also shares clinical vignettes and helpful information to group leaders who are working with this vulnerable population. Dr. Kanas reminds us of the heart and soul of these patients who benefit from todays' treatment and the power of group therapy to facilitate change."

Cheri L. Marmarosh, PhD, Associate Professor of
Professional Psychology, George Washington University;
Fellow, American Psychology Association; Associate Editor of
Psychotherapy; and on the editorial boards of *Group Dynamics:*
Theory, Research, and Practice and the *International*
Journal of Group Psychotherapy; Fellow, American Group
Psychotherapy Association

"As a clinical psychologist who has spent nearly four decades doing both group and individual therapy with non-psychotic patients, and teaching/supervising numerous psychiatrists and psychologists to do so as well, I was surprised by how clearly and simply Dr. Kanas could provide a model for working with a group of patients for which I had so little training and experience. Unlike my anticipation that I would find that there was too much new here to be either readily or usefully absorbed, I found the book to be a terrific mini-course on the nature of psychosis and to provide an easily learnable evidence-based approach to effective treatment. In short, though I had expected this book to be a challenging and perhaps exhausting workout, I found it to be surprisingly enjoyable, highly readable, and of great potential value to anyone involved in the treatment of mental illness—especially to those working with psychotic patients."

Geraldine Alpert, PhD, Past President of the Northern
California Group Psychotherapy Society; former Director of
Group Therapy Training, McAuley Neuropsychiatric
Institute; Associate Clinical Professor of Psychiatry,
University of California Medical School; Fellow, American
Group Psychotherapy Association

Integrative Group Therapy for Psychosis

An Evidence-Based Approach

Nick Kanas

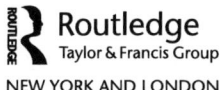

Routledge
Taylor & Francis Group

NEW YORK AND LONDON

First published 2021
by Routledge
52 Vanderbilt Avenue, New York, NY 10017

and by Routledge
2 Park Square, Milton Park, Abingdon, Oxon, OX14 4RN

Routledge is an imprint of the Taylor & Francis Group, an informa business

© 2021 Taylor & Francis

Library of Congress Cataloging-in-Publication Data
Names: Kanas, Nick, 1945- author.
Title: Integrative group therapy for psychosis: an evidence-based
approach / Nick Kanas.
Description: New York, NY: Routledge, 2021. | Includes
bibliographical references and index.
Identifiers: LCCN 2020013789 (print) | LCCN 2020013790 (ebook) |
ISBN 9780367340391 (hardback) | ISBN 9780367339425 (paperback) |
ISBN 9781003056553 (ebook)
Subjects: MESH: Psychotic Disorders—therapy | Psychotherapy,
Group—methods | Integrative Medicine | Evidence-Based Medicine
Classification: LCC RC454 (print) | LCC RC454 (ebook) |
NLM WM 200 | DDC 616.89—dc23
LC record available at https://lccn.loc.gov/2020013789
LC ebook record available at https://lccn.loc.gov/2020013790

ISBN: 978-0-367-34039-1 (hbk)
ISBN: 978-0-367-33942-5 (pbk)
ISBN: 978-1-003-05655-3 (ebk)

Typeset in Times New Roman
by codeMantra

For my wife Carolynn, who has been a great support on life's journey with me for more than four decades, and as a psychiatric nurse encouraged me to write this book for the benefit of patients learning to cope with their psychotic disorder.

Contents

List of Tables   x
List of Figures   xii
Author Biography   xiii
Preface   xiv
Acknowledgement   xvi

1   Nature of Psychotic Conditions   1

2   Historical and Clinical Issues   16

3   Research Issues   60

4   Clinical Issues of the Integrative Model: The Basics   76

5   Clinical Issues of the Integrative Model: Special Topics   114

6   Evaluation of the Integrative Model   127

7   Integrative Groups for Non-Psychotic Bipolar Patients   145

8   Conclusions   174

Index   179

Tables

1.1 Characteristics of psychosis 4

1.2 Thought disorders 10

2.1 Bellak's 12 ego functions in schizophrenia 23

2.2 Attachment styles (according to Marmarosh, Markin and Spiegel, 2013) 25

2.3 Attachment styles (according to Wickham, Sitko and Bentall, 2015) 26

3.1 Effectiveness of group therapy for schizophrenic patients: number (%) of studies 62

3.2 Influence of clinical category on group therapy effectiveness: proportion (%) of groups 63

4.1 Integrative model: psychodynamic issues 79

4.2 Integrative model: interpersonal issues 82

4.3 Integrative model: cognitive-behavioral issues 84

4.4 Integrative model: psychoeducational issues 87

4.5 Group format issues: integrative groups 95

4.6 Effects of setting and group developmental history on group goals 99

4.7 Examples of discussion topics 103

4.8 Examples of coping strategies 106

4.9 Tips for the therapist 108

6.1 Ranking of therapeutic factors in a short-term inpatient group (Kanas and Barr, 1982) 130

6.2 HIM-G category percentile scores for integrative groups versus normative groups 131

6.3 GCQ-S mean dimension scores 132

6.4 Ranking of therapeutic factors in a short-term outpatient group (Kanas et al., 1988) 136

6.5 Significant follow-up dimension scores: group versus control patients (Kanas et al., 1989a) 137

6.6 Ranking of therapeutic factors in a long-term outpatient group 140

7.1 Goals of integrative group therapy for non-psychotic bipolar patients 158

7.2 Discussion topics in integrative group therapy
for non-psychotic bipolar patients 161
7.3 Differences between integrative psychosis groups and
non-psychosis bipolar groups 163
7.4 Group format issues: non-psychosis bipolar groups 165

Figures

6.1   Integrative Group Outcome and Process Questionnaire   129

Author Biography

Dr. Kanas is an Emeritus Professor of Psychiatry at the University of California, San Francisco (UCSF). He trained at Stanford University (B.A. Psychology), University of California, Los Angeles, Medical School (M.D. 1971), University of Texas Medical Branch in Galveston (Internship), and UCSF (Psychiatry Residency 1975). After training and serving in the USAF as a psychiatrist, he joined the faculty at UCSF and the affiliated San Francisco Department of Veterans Affairs Medical Center, where he conducted clinical and research work on people suffering from stressful conditions. He directed the Group Therapy Training Program for the UCSF department of psychiatry. He is a fellow of the American Group Psychotherapy Association, wrote a book entitled *Group Therapy for Schizophrenic Patients*, and continues to edit the Research Reviews section of the *International Journal of Group Psychotherapy*. He has over 215 professional publications and is the recipient of the Dr. J. Elliott Royer Award for academic psychiatry. You are holding his latest group therapy book entitled: *Integrative Group Therapy for Psychosis: An Evidence-Based Approach*.

Since 1970, he has studied and written about psychological and interpersonal issues affecting people living and working in space. He has done space-related research since the late 1980s, and for over 15 years, he was a NASA-funded principal investigator, doing psychological research with astronauts and cosmonauts. He is a member and former trustee of the International Academy of Astronautics, and he has been a consultant to private aerospace companies. Together with Dietrich Manzey, he is the coauthor of the textbook entitled *Space Psychology and Psychiatry, 2nd ed.*, which was given the 2004 International Academy of Astronautics Life Science Book Award. In 1999, Dr. Kanas received the Aerospace Medical Association Raymond F. Longacre Award for Outstanding Accomplishment in the Psychological and Psychiatric Aspects of Aerospace Medicine. In 2008, he received the International Academy of Astronautics Life Science Award. His latest book on space psychology, entitled *Humans in Space: The Psychological Hurdles*, was given the 2016 International Academy of Astronautics Life Science Book Award.

For more on Dr. Kanas's books, including his celestial map books and his science fiction novels, visit his website: **www.nickkanas.com**.

Preface

This book is an updated and expanded version of my previous book entitled: *Group Therapy for Schizophrenic Patients* (1996). It was in this earlier work that I first used the term *integrative* to describe the treatment model, which had been developed empirically via several outcome and process research studies. Although much of the treatment model presented in the earlier book has remained the same over the years, there are some new developments.

First, I have been leading and studying therapy groups for schizophrenic patients continuously since 1975, more than 45 years. I also have authored and coauthored numerous research papers published in peer-reviewed journals, and I have presented open sessions and workshops on this topic at annual meetings of the American Group Psychotherapy Association since the 1980s. In addition, I have edited the Research Reviews section of the *International Journal of Group Psychotherapy* since 1999. All of these activities have put me in a position to appreciate the importance of coordinating research findings and clinical practice in group therapy;hence, the title of the current volume: *Integrative Group Therapy for Psychosis: An Evidence-Based Approach*. In keeping with current evidence-based requirements of clinical work, this new book incorporates the latest research findings involving therapy groups with psychotic patients to defend both the general approach and the specifics of my integrative model, especially in Chapters 3 and 6. In addition, research findings are presented for non-psychosis bipolar groups in Chapter 7. Therapy groups continue to be underutilized in psychosis, and it is my hope that the overwhelming empirical support for this treatment model will turn the tide.

Second, my previous book on this topic emphasized the integration of psychodynamic, interpersonal, and psychoeducational theory and techniques, with the latter incorporating some elements from cognitive-behavior therapy (CBT). Over the years, CBT has expanded as a form of group therapy, with much research support showing its effectiveness. Many of these newer CBT approaches have been incorporated into my model, and I felt the need to be more explicit in describing them. So, the updated model presented in this book highlights four approaches integrated into one: psychodynamic, interpersonal, psychoeducational, and cognitive-behavioral.

Third, the scope of this book has been expanded over the previous book, which mainly focused on patients with schizophrenia. The approach described here covers a broader range of patients who have chronic psychotic symptoms as a common feature. In addition, Chapter 7 deals with a modification of the basic integrative model specifically designed for non-psychotic bipolar patients, whose needs during their euthymic periods are different than those of more floridly psychotic patients.

Finally, this book expands upon the clinical material presented in the earlier work, with numerous tables, two group therapy session descriptions, 26 clinical group vignettes illustrating key points, and several excerpts from a book written by a licensed clinical social worker describing his battle with schizophrenia. This clinical material forms the basis of Chapters 1, 2, 4, and 5 as well as Chapter 7 for non-psychotic bipolar patients. It is my hope that this book will be a guide for psychiatrists, psychologists, social workers, nurses, and other mental health professionals and students who treat patients with schizophrenia spectrum disorders and other psychoses as well as non-psychotic bipolar disorder. The integrative group therapy treatment model presented here is meant to be an important adjunct to psychoactive medications that will help these patients learn more about their illness and develop strategies of coping with its debilitating symptoms.

Reference

Kanas, N. (1996) *Group Therapy for Schizophrenic Patients*. Washington, DC: American Psychiatric Press.

Acknowledgement

I would like to thank Robert Francis (pen name) for giving me permission to quote some of his experiences from his book *On Conquering Schizophrenia: From the Desk of a Therapist and Survivor, with Purview on Metaphysics, Philosophy, and Theology* (2019). As a licensed clinical social worker who also suffers from chronic schizophrenia, his insights bring home the reality and pain of this disorder in a way that both lay and professional people can understand. I recommend this book for anyone interested in a first-hand account of the schizophrenic experience.

Reference

Francis, R. (2019) *On Conquering Schizophrenia: From the Desk of a Therapist and Survivor, with Purview on Metaphysics, Philosophy, and Theology.* Bloomington, IN: iUniverse Press.

1 Nature of Psychotic Conditions

Introduction

People with psychosis have severe thinking and mood impairments that cause them to lose contact with external reality. These impairments may affect belief systems, perceptions, thought processes, behaviors, motivations, emotional states, and relationships with other people. Most psychotic individuals experience or sense reality differently from others, and they have an impaired ability to test the validity of their experiences.

Under certain conditions, anyone can experience a transient psychosis. For example, as a young medical student, who had been on-call with no sleep for 36 hours, I once had the experience of hearing someone call my name while walking down a long hallway. I looked around and didn't see anyone. I laughed to myself and said: "Boy, I need to get some sleep" and went home for a nap. Although my reality sense was temporarily impaired by lack of sleep, my reality testing ability was intact, and I was able to dismiss the voices as due to sleep deprivation. In contrast, a psychotic individual would believe in the reality of his or her hallucinations and might even conjure up a delusional belief as an explanation rather than simply looking around and, not seeing anyone, pass them off as a production of the mind.

Etiology and Psychopathology of Psychosis

Genetic and developmental factors play a big role in psychotic conditions (Sadock, Sadock and Ruiz, 2009a). For example, in schizophrenia, monozygotic twins have a concordance rate of 50% for the disease, and in bipolar disorder, this jumps to about 70%. As worldwide problems, schizophrenia affects about 0.5% of the population at a given time. For the mood disorders, psychiatric researcher Hagop Akiskal believes that better detection of bipolar II disorder has raised the point prevalence number for these conditions. He has stated that

> the conventional figure of 1 percent for bipolar disorders in the general population is being challenged, and there are now convincing

data that this group of disorders may account for 5 percent of the population and up to 50 percent of all depressions.

(Sadock, Sadock and Ruiz, 2009a, p. 1629)

External stressors (e.g., lack of sleep, life-threatening events) and physiological factors (e.g., drugs, medications, medical illnesses) also may precipitate a psychotic episode.

Specific neurodevelopmental and neurocognitive deficits have been found to occur in psychotic patients, especially those suffering from schizophrenia (Sadock, Sadock and Ruiz, 2009a). Beck and Rector (2005) point to neuroimaging and other evidence to suggest that many people with schizophrenia have pathological changes in their brains, such as enlarged lateral ventricles and abnormalities in their hippocampus and prefrontal lobes. The resulting cognitive deficits may be found early in childhood and often precede the advent of other disease characteristics; they may be more significant determinants of functional outcome in work, school, and daily living than positive symptoms (e.g., hallucinations, delusions) or negative symptoms (e.g., decreased emotional responses, lack of motivation); and they usually do not improve during periods of remission (Hurford, Kalkstein and Hurford, 2011; Vinogradov, 2019). Cognitive and brain changes also have been found in psychological tests, leading to deficits in executive functions, attention, speed of processing auditory and visual information, learning (including socially relevant information), and memory (especially verbal memory) (Beck and Rector, 2005; Hurford, Kalkstein and Hurford, 2011; Nuechterlein and Dawson, 1984; Vinogradov, 2019).

There is strong evidence that negative symptoms especially are related to structural changes in the brains of schizophrenic patients. For example, the results from one study concluded that patients with schizophrenia who had especially large ventricles suffered from diffuse brain abnormalities (mainly atrophic), impaired cognitive functioning, and a preponderance of negative symptoms, while patients with the smallest ventricles were characterized by more focal brain dysfunction (primarily neurochemical), a normal sensorium, and a preponderance of positive symptoms (Andreasen et al., 1982). Negative symptoms have shown a higher concordance rate in monozygotic twins than positive symptoms, suggesting a greater genetic influence (Dworkin and Lenzenweger, 1984). These findings point to a strong biological predisposition to the development of negative symptoms that may begin premorbidly with cognitive beliefs of low expectancies for pleasure and success, a perception of having limited resources, and negative attitudes toward social affiliation and acceptance by others. This may account for the high prevalence of premorbid avoidant, schizoid, paranoid, dependent, and schizotypal personality disorders found in schizophrenia (Solano and De Chavez, 2000). Some negative symptoms also may be a secondary reaction to positive symptoms. For example, persecutory delusions may lead to avoidance of other people who may be a threat, or unbidden auditory hallucinations may lead to a sense of not having control over one's thoughts and a need to withdraw and conserve resources.

Early on, the psychotic state may be latent, and people with this condition may simply be seen as odd or eccentric. Later on, a life event or no apparent cause may result in an acute psychotic episode that requires hospitalization. Sometimes, psychotic symptoms may simmer into a more chronic pattern that becomes worse over time. In all cases, psychosis may negatively affect a person's ability to work, care for him- or herself, and relate with other people. When the predominant deficiency is in the area of thinking, we speak of a thought disorder, such as schizophrenia or delusional disorder. When the predominant deficiency is in the area of emotions, we speak of a mood disorder, such as bipolar disorder or major depression.

Treatment of Psychosis

The treatment for psychosis includes biological, psychological, and social components.

In the biological realm, this usually means medications. These range from antipsychotic medications for people with thought disorders (such as schizophrenia spectrum disorders) to antidepressants for people with depression to lithium and mood stabilizers for people with bipolar disorder (Preston and Johnson, 2019; Preston, O'Neal and Talaga, 2017). Electroconvulsive therapy also may be used to treat medication-resistant patients with a mood disorder.

Medications usually are prescribed by physicians in an office, a separate clinic, or a medication group (Stone, 1996). Sometimes, they are prescribed after a psychotherapy session by the therapist if he or she happens to be a psychiatrist. In such a case, it is important to not overlap the therapy and prescribing activities during the same session.

Although medications are very important in treating psychosis, they are not enough. As Stone has stated:

> A schizophrenic adult, who because of peculiarities as a child was shunned or ridiculed and as a consequence did not develop the interpersonal relationships either inside or outside of the family that might sustain or support him or her, will not have problems solved with medications, even those that hold promise to improve negative symptoms of the illness.
>
> (Stone, 1996, p. vii)

Supportive individual and family therapy may be indicated for psychological issues, and there is evidence that psychotic individuals spend less time in the hospital when psychotherapy is added to medications in the treatment plan (Martindale et al., 2000).

In the social realm, adequate housing, financial support, and recreational and occupational therapy may be indicated. For acutely disturbed patients, hospitalization may be necessary until they can be stabilized and prepared for outpatient treatment. Many psychotic patients have a co-occurring substance use disorder, which complicates their treatment (Horsfall et al., 2009).

What about group therapy? While beneficial for people suffering from non-psychotic conditions, how useful is it for people suffering from psychosis? At first thought, it would seem that a talk-oriented therapy would not be terribly helpful for people with breaks in reality. However, as we shall see in the next two chapters, the literature suggests otherwise and supports group therapy as part of a biopsychosocial treatment plan. But first, let's examine the characteristics of psychosis more fully.

DSM-5 Criteria for the Psychoses

Formal diagnosis is a useful way to set up therapy groups with psychotic patients. In this book, I will use the standardized criteria described in the American Psychiatric Association *Diagnostic and Statistical Manual of Mental Disorders, Fifth Edition,* commonly abbreviated as DSM-5 (2013). In this system, psychosis is characterized by abnormalities in one or more of the five domains shown in Table 1.1. These will be described in the sections below.

To enliven these descriptions, I will insert some excerpts from a remarkable book entitled *On Conquering Schizophrenia: From the Desk of a Therapist and Survivor, with Purview on Metaphysics, Philosophy, and Theology* by Robert Francis. As the first part of the subtitle indicates, Mr. Francis (a pen name) is a person suffering from chronic schizophrenia and also

Table 1.1 Characteristics of psychosis

Domain	Definition
Delusions	Fixed, unrealistic beliefs not amenable to change in light of conflicting evidence
Hallucinations	Perception-like experiences that occur in the absence of an external stimulus
Disorganized thinking/ speech	Confused thought associations that are severe enough to impair communications
Disorganized or abnormal motor behavior	Bizarre physical movements or marked decreased reactivity to the environment (catatonia)
Negative symptoms	Decreased emotional responses to people or lack of motivation to engage in purposeful activity

licensed and employed as a social worker. In college, he received a B.A. in communications with a minor in philosophy, which accounts for the second part of the subtitle. In fact, the beginning and ending chapters of the book contain his musings on philosophy and religion. But the central chapters contain vivid descriptions of his psychotic symptoms. He began experiencing these symptoms at about age 21 and was subsequently diagnosed as having "schizophrenia, paranoid type." After some rough years, he managed to learn strategies of coping with his symptoms, and in his early 30s, he went back to school and obtained his master's degree in social work. Now in his 40s, he has worked as a Licensed Clinical Social Worker conducting therapy in the fields of mental health and in substance abuse. Quotes from his book are given below.

According to the DSM-5 (2013), delusions are fixed beliefs that have little or no basis in reality. There are several kinds: persecutory (beliefs that one is going to be harmed by an individual or group), referential (beliefs that certain gestures, comments, etc. are directed at oneself), somatic (beliefs about unsupportable physical problems), religious (beliefs not supported by an organized religious group), grandiose (beliefs that one has exceptional abilities or fame), jealousy (irrational beliefs that a spouse or lover is unfaithful), erotomanic (beliefs that another person is in love with you with no basis in fact), and nihilistic (beliefs that a major catastrophe is imminent). In addition, the DSM-5 recognizes certain clearly implausible delusions as bizarre (e.g., beliefs that someone has removed or altered one's internal organs, or that one's thoughts have been removed or inserted by an outside force, or that one's actions are controlled by an external agency).

Francis (2019) says this about some of his delusions:

> When I am under the influence or persuasion of a delusion, clinically speaking, I am experiencing and projecting a current belief about the specific situation, myself, or others that is in stark contrast to the larger tacitly agreed upon mutually socially constructed reality of the masses…A specific grandiose delusion I once experienced was that I was in a friendship with the then President of the United States. This delusion was recurrent over time and was intermittent over a period of many years…such delusions have been far more infrequent compared to other types of delusions, especially the type known as persecutory delusions…These types of delusions can be brief in time, can last minutes to hours, or can be more perseverative spanning days, weeks, months, or even years…Persecutory delusions are marked by beliefs that others are deliberately trying to cause pain, suffering, humiliation, fear, and harm to me…Oftentimes, in my experience, the delusions are perceptions of a pure form of evil intent.
>
> (Francis, 2019, pp. 40–41)

He goes on to describe the various types of persecutory delusions he has had, such as:

> ...being used by the federal government in a manipulative ploy, having a microchip implanted in my brain when sleeping in order to control me, lobotomized while asleep, being abducted by aliens and physically transplanted onto a different planet, being rejected by all other people including family as well as being rejected by God, believing others know all of my thoughts..., contemplations of actually being present in "Hell," the belief of being captured on live video for the rest of humanity to observe, and the belief that I am under remote control by others.
>
> (Francis, 2019, p. 42)

Although frightening, his ability to cope with these delusions over time altered their impact:

> Early in my illness, these types of delusions triggered me to behave in a highly erratic and irrational manners (sic), and triggered intense feelings of utter hopelessness. Over the course of my illness, although still very arduous and challenging, managing such delusions is a bit less difficult due to their increasing familiarity and my increasing insight. Twenty some odd years into my illness the delusion of the microchip, for example, does not bother me as much as it once did. When I experience the recurrent microchip delusion, I now say to myself, for example and in part, that the microchip is a "possibility." And because of its recurrence and its now modest familiarity, I retort to myself that even if it is true, "I really do not care anymore."
>
> (Francis, 2019, p. 43)

According to DSM-5, hallucinations are associated with the five senses and so are perceived as being auditory, visual, tactile or somatic, gustatory, or olfactory. They usually are experienced as being vivid and clear and not under voluntary control. Auditory hallucinations are most common in schizophrenia and related conditions, and they usually are perceived as being distinct from one's thoughts (i.e., voices or sounds coming from the outside). There are no stimuli-prompting hallucinations, unlike illusions (e.g., perceiving a table with four legs as an animal with four legs). Some hallucinations are considered as being common and normal, such as those that occur when falling asleep (hypnagogic hallucinations) or waking up (hypnopompic hallucinations) or those that are part of a culturally sanctioned religious experience (e.g., hearing God speak to a congregation).

Francis (2019) says this about his auditory hallucinations:

> Usually, the voices I hear sound as coming from the external environment rather than internally from my own mind. The voices are

mostly horrifying and disturbing and are persistently derogatory and often penetrate my vulnerabilities...The voices can be frequent, intermittent, and/or occasional. In my experience, the content of the hallucinations oftentimes presents as the worst possible thing to be heard for that particular moment and for that particular situation... An interesting aspect to my auditory hallucinations is that after hearing the voice for a period they begin to integrate into my mind as parcel to my own cognitive functioning.

(Francis, 2019, pp. 39–40)

For Francis, auditory hallucinations and persecutory delusions can occur together and often are accompanied by feelings of paranoia, which he describes as follows:

The feeling is not of being a little suspicious or a little ill at ease, rather, it is much more profound and encompassing...In my experience, paranoia is a feeling that is dark and horrifying, and perhaps most importantly, a feeling marked by hopelessness. It is a feeling of pervasive doom, and even at times a feeling of being, as a matter of fact, eternally damned...The feeling can persist over time for hours, days, and sometimes months. It is a state of mind conducive to suicidality.

(Francis, 2019, p. 39)

Disorganized thinking is a problem that involves the process of thought. It can be discovered simply by listening to a person's uninterrupted flow of speech. Switching from one topic to an unrelated topic is called loose associations, connecting one topic to another via a secondary association is called tangentiality, circling around a theme before finally coming to a point is called circumstantial thinking, and speech that is completely incoherent is called word salad. Some people exhibit mild and transient disorganized speech when they are socially anxious or unclear about a concept they are trying to explain. Also, people with acute organic brain syndrome due to drugs or medical illness can exhibit disorganized thinking. To be considered a symptom of psychosis, the disorganization should be nonlinear and severe enough to impair communication with others.

Francis (2019) seems to accept nonlinear thinking as a philosophical given when he discusses his notion of ideas:

In my mind, ideas are much too beautiful to bludgeoned (sic) in total into a comprehensively linear and mechanical form. Ideas by their vary nature are nonlinear, non-chronological, and more of a conglomeration of thoughts united by common themes. Ideas connect a number of thoughts that superficially may have no connection. I view ideas similarly to Plato's conception of the "**forms**." I see ideas as ideals.

(Francis, 2019, pp. 49–50)

But for the sake of the reader of his book and with good humor, he returns to "regular programming" by continuing his narrative in linear fashion!

In the DSM-5, grossly disorganized or abnormal motor behavior may vary from childish silliness to unpredictable agitation that impairs the ability to perform normal activities of daily life or any other goal-directed behavior. This includes catatonia, which is a marked decrease in reactivity to the environment, ranging from resistance to instructions (negativism), to rigid or bizarre posturing, to complete lack of verbal and motor responses (mutism and stupor). Repeated stereotyped movements and echoing of speech also may occur. Sometimes, psychotic people exhibit unexpected explosive and purposeless motor activity (catatonic excitement).

Negative symptoms are more prominent in people with schizophrenia than in other psychotic conditions, especially diminished emotional expression (as manifested by decreased facial and hand movements, eye contact, and intonation of speech) and avolition (as manifested by decreased motivation for or engagement in self-initiated purposeful activities). Other examples of negative symptoms include diminished speech output (alogia), decreased ability to experience pleasure in positive situations (anhedonia), and lack of interest in pursuing social interactions (asociality).

Describing his negative symptoms in general terms, Francis (2019) says the following:

> My experience of the negative symptoms mostly feels like a statically low mood that feels resistant to change, along with pervasive and lasting feelings of a psychic nothingness. The felt experience of the negative symptoms seems to mostly occur when the positive symptoms abate for the time being. During these time periods, my thought content seems to drain and empty of the frenetic and energetic pathological positive symptoms as I transition into the dulling abyss of the negative symptoms.
>
> (Francis, 2019, p. 52)

Francis further discusses negative symptoms in terms of problems with affect and with amotivation to do things. He defines affect as one's generalized background emotional climate, and he contrasts it with mood, which is more an acute, current emotional state. One affective problem he discusses is incongruency, which he says:

> ... is a descriptor used to indicate a mismatch between what is being spoken and the corresponding underlying mood that comes with the spoken content...The most important aspect about incongruent affect in my experience is that it is not a symptom, in and of itself,

that is particularly distressing much like the others. An incongruent affect is more of a clinical indicator of an existing thought disorder rather than an experientially distressing specified symptom.

(Francis, 2019, pp. 50–51)

Another affect problem is being flat, which "is characterized by a statically expressionless drawn and sullen face" (Francis, 2019, p. 51). He associates flat affect with poverty of thought and poverty of speech and says:

In the experience of my "schizo" illness, all three of these symptoms have at one time or another been active. To this day, I cannot elude an affective flatness. I behaviorally compensate when in a social context but when alone there is no escape...I feel substantially "zoned out," mildly depressed, and it causes me to want to isolate and not be around others.

(Francis, 2019, p. 52)

These symptoms also lead to thought blocking, which he experiences as:

...a state of having no flow or succession to one's thoughts...there is a pervasive feel of a cognitive nothingness...Its primary effect is that it inhibits my communication abilities...It is the analogous equivalent of your brain being stuck in concrete.

(Francis, 2019, p. 52)

Francis defines the negative symptom of amotivation as "a generalized lack of gainful activity" (2019, p. 52) that can affect regular work and social actions and can lead to a sedentary life. It can even affect basic activities of daily living, such as proper hygiene. Since he forces himself to be active every day, he feels that amotivation is low on his list of problems.

Note that several of these negative symptoms directly impact on forming interpersonal relationships, and all of them indirectly cause problems in interacting with other people. Psychotic people have problems dealing with the reality of the world, and for human beings, this includes their social reality. Any treatment of people with psychosis must consider ways of helping them deal with others, either in terms of meeting and casually interacting in social contexts or in forming deeper relationships that last over time.

Broadly speaking, one can divide psychotic conditions into two kinds: thought disorders, where the primary problem deals with the process and content of thoughts and cognitions, and mood disorders, where the primary problem is in the emotional area but where extreme highs or lows can affect a person's belief about him- or herself, other people, or the world at large to a psychotic degree. Let's look at these two domains.

Thought Disorders

In DSM-5 terms, thought disorders largely are categorized as "Schizophrenia Spectrum and Other Psychotic Disorders," and most of these are listed in Table 1.2. In this book, I will include delusional disorder in the schizophrenia spectrum of diseases (i.e., the first six rows in Table 1.2), since all share similar phenomenological and treatment implications.

Schizotypal disorder is actually a personality disorder. It is included here because people with this condition have symptoms similar to those in Table 1.1, but to a lesser degree. They have a pattern of social and interpersonal deficits and cognitive or perceptual distortions that include five or more of the following symptoms: ideas of reference not reaching a delusional degree; odd beliefs or magical thinking (telepathy, clairvoyance); bodily illusions and other perceptual distortions; odd thinking or speech (metaphorical, overelaborate, stereotyped); general suspiciousness of others; inappropriate or constricted affect; peculiar behaviors; lack of close friends; and excessive social anxiety.

People with delusional disorder are characterized by having at least one month of delusions but no other psychotic symptoms; although in some cases, hallucinations may occur that are related to the delusional theme (e.g., feeling insects in the body consistent with delusions of infestation). The delusions may evolve into a complicated, internally consistent system, and general functioning and behavior may not generally be seen as impaired by outside observers. Note that with this condition and in other conditions mentioned below with duration criteria, the time course may be affected by successful treatment with psychotherapy or medications.

Brief psychotic disorders are characterized by episodes of at least one of the following lasting at least one day but less than one month: delusions, hallucinations, disorganized speech, or grossly disorganized or

Table 1.2 Thought disorders

Schizotypal (personality) disorder
Delusional disorder
Brief psychotic disorder
Schizophreniform disorder
Schizophrenia
Schizoaffective disorder
Substance/medication-induced psychotic disorder
Psychotic disorder due to another medical condition
Catatonia associated with another mental disorder (catatonia specifier)
Catatonia due to another medical condition
Unspecified catatonia
Unspecified schizophrenia spectrum and other psychotic disorder
Other specified schizophrenia spectrum and other psychotic disorder

catatonic behavior. These people usually return to premorbid levels of functioning after the episode abates.

Schizophreniform disorders have episodes with two or more of the following lasting at least one month but less than six months: delusions, hallucinations, disorganized speech, grossly disorganized or catatonic behavior, or negative symptoms.

Schizophrenia lasts for at least six months and includes at least a one-month period of active-phase symptoms and signs similar to those of schizophreniform disorder. But in addition, subsequent to the onset of the disorder, there needs to be a decline in level of functioning in work, school, interpersonal relations, or self-care as well as residual symptoms and signs described in the active phase but in an attenuated form (e.g., odd beliefs, unusual perceptual experiences).

In schizoaffective disorder, a mood episode (see below) and the active-phase symptoms and signs of schizophrenia occur together. In addition, these are preceded or followed by at least two weeks of delusions or hallucinations without prominent mood symptoms.

The above psychotic conditions are primary, in that they are not related to taking drugs or medications or part of non-psychiatric medical conditions. In contrast, substance or medication-induced psychotic disorders are a physiological consequence of exposure to a drug of abuse, a medication, or a toxin. Such agents can cause hallucinations, delusions, or delirium, either during the exposure or, for some agents, withdrawal from the drug. Impairment in social, occupational, or other areas of functioning occurs. Symptoms usually remit after the offending agent is removed from the body. Stimulants, such as amphetamines or cocaine, and hallucinogens especially are prone to cause psychosis, but any drug or medication can have psychotic effects, depending on its actions and dosage. The same may be said for psychotic disorders due to non-psychiatric medical conditions, such as thyroid disease, brain tumor, or endocrine malfunction.

Like delusional disorder, catatonia per se is defined in the absence of other psychotic symptoms or signs. It is characterized by marked psychomotor disturbance ranging from marked unresponsiveness to marked agitation to bizarre movements. The DSM-5 states that three or more of the following need to be present for full-blown catatonia: stupor, catalepsy (passive induction of a posture held against gravity), posturing (spontaneous and active maintenance of a posture against gravity), waxy flexibility (slight, even resistance to positioning by the examiner), mutism, negativism, mannerism (odd caricatures of normal actions), stereotypy (repetitive, abnormally frequent movements that are non-goal directed), agitation, grimacing, echolalia (mimicking other's speech), and echopraxia (mimicking other's movements). Since catatonic symptoms can occur as part of another psychiatric disorder (e.g., schizophrenia, bipolar, or depressive disorder), if there is marked psychomotor disturbance and if three of the above clinical signs are present, it should be coded as being associated with another mental disorder as a catatonia specifier. Catatonia also may be caused by a non-psychiatric medical condition (e.g., cerebral folate deficiency, certain autoimmune and paraneoplastic disorders) or as a side effect of a medication.

Sometimes, a psychotic condition does not meet all of the criteria for one of the above psychiatric disorders or there is inadequate or contradictory information presented to the clinician (such as might occur in an emergency room). Such conditions can be subsumed as unspecified catatonia or unspecified schizophrenia spectrum and other psychotic disorder. Occasionally, there are specific psychotic-like symptoms that are present that dominate the clinical picture but do not exactly match the criteria for one of the above psychotic conditions. Examples include persistent auditory hallucinations in the absence of other psychotic features, delusions with significant overlapping mood episodes, attenuated psychotic syndrome with symptoms below the threshold for full psychosis, or delusional symptoms reinforced by a relationship with a dominant psychotic partner (such as can happen in *folie à deux*). In DSM-5, such cases can be diagnosed as "other specified schizophrenia spectrum and other psychotic disorder," followed by the specific features used to make the diagnosis.

Mood Disorders

The DSM-5 recognizes two distinct classes of mood disorder: bipolar I and II and related disorders (which may include depressive episodes) and depressive disorders (which don't usually include manic episodes). In both groups, psychotic symptoms may be a part of the syndrome but are not necessary to make the diagnosis for all patients. For example, to make the diagnosis of bipolar I disorder, three of seven symptoms and signs characteristic of a manic episode are necessary. Three of the latter may reach psychotic proportions: inflated self-esteem or grandiosity (delusion), flight of ideas or racing thoughts (disorganized thinking), and pressured tangential speech (disorganized speech). Most acute manic individuals experience such psychotic symptoms. Many of these people also undergo a major depressive episode, which may include feelings of worthlessness or inappropriate guilt that may reach delusional proportions. People also experience major depressive episodes without a manic or hypomanic component, but again their negative view of themselves may reach psychotic proportions. Bipolar and depressive disorders may arise on their own or be induced by drugs, medications, and medical conditions. More will be said about bipolar disorders in Chapter 7.

As opposed to some of the thought disorders described above (e.g., delusional disorder, schizophrenia), where elements of psychosis persist after the active phase of the illness, psychotic symptoms and signs tend to go away after the acute phases of bipolar I and II and depressive disorders.

What remains is a constant battle to corral emotions and guard against the recurrence of an acute episode. However, some of these individuals have a persistent and unrealistic sense of self-esteem (either too low or too high) and pacing of their thoughts (either too slow or too fast), depending on whether they are depressed or hypomanic. Such symptoms dip into psychosis and remain problematic for these individuals. In addition, many of these people are bright and can function at a high level when not acutely ill. However, the frequency of devastating manic or depressive episodes, and the residual symptoms that continue when they are not acutely ill (the euthymic state), can retard their work momentum and interfere with their interpersonal relationships, which may further lower their self-esteem.

Other Psychotic-Like Conditions

There are other conditions that may result in transient psychotic-like symptoms. For example, people undergoing a dissociative disorder (e.g., depersonalization/derealization disorder) may feel detached from their body or mental processes (depersonalization) or feel that their surroundings are unreal (derealization). Although reality sense is impaired, reality testing ability usually is intact, and these people rarely have other symptoms characteristic of psychosis.

People with a stress-related disorder (e.g., posttraumatic stress disorder, acute stress disorder) also may experience depersonalization or derealization. If the stressor is unusually intense, hallucinations and delusions may occur. In this case, we may be speaking of a brief psychotic disorder or brief reactive psychosis. Such a condition also may occur to a person not otherwise diagnosed with a mental disorder but who is undergoing extreme stress (justifying the military expression that "every man has his breaking point").

People with borderline personality disorder also may experience transient stress-related paranoid ideation or severe dissociative symptoms. They also can experience unstable interpersonal relationships, problems with their self-image, and real or imagined abandonment. Although rarely psychotic in the absence of stress, these individuals typically get themselves in compromising situations, and high stress may be a part of their lives.

Other Diagnostic Systems

Although this book will follow the APA diagnostic system, mention will be made of three other classification approaches (Sadock, Sadock and Ruiz, 2009a). The first is the *International Classification of Diseases, 10th Ed., Classification of Mental and Behavioural Disorders* (World Health Organization, 1992) or ICD-10. Although the DSM-5 is used in America and several other countries, the ICD-10 was developed for international use and still is popular in places like Russia and China. Both systems have a high degree of concordance in terms of psychotic conditions, however. Two major differences for schizophrenia are that the DSM-5 requires a duration of six months and deterioration in social and occupational function for a diagnosis, whereas the ICD-10 requires only one month and no need for socio-occupational deterioration for a diagnosis. But the basic symptomologies are very similar.

Historically, the various classification systems of mood and thought disorders are extensive and varied and beyond the scope of this book. The interested reader is referred to a standard textbook such as Sadock, Sadock and Ruiz (2009a, b). However, I will mention briefly the work of two neuropsychiatrists who had an impact on the field of schizophrenia that still has relevance for today. Eugen Bleuler (1857–1959) proposed the term "schizophrenia" in 1911 to denote his view of a splitting of psychic functions. He identified four primary symptoms of the disorder: abnormal or *loose associations*, *autistic* thinking and behavior, inappropriate *affect*, and *ambivalence*. For decades thereafter, Bleuler's "4 A's" were viewed as the defining criteria of the disease, and older clinicians still think about these criteria as a short-hand method for making a diagnosis. Bleuler viewed hallucinations, delusions, and social withdrawal as secondary manifestations of the illness that were affected by the adaptive capacity of the patient and environmental circumstances. These criteria are given primary relevance in the DSM-5 and ICD-10 systems.

Kurt Schneider (1887–1967) focused on various symptoms of schizophrenia as the defining characteristics of the illness. His "first rank" symptoms were composed of a variety of hallucinations, delusions, and characteristics of thinking. Examples included: audible thoughts coming from outside one's head (auditory hallucinations); voices arguing or commenting on a patient's actions; tactile or visceral hallucinations caused by an outside agent; thoughts being removed or inserted into one's mind (thought withdrawal or insertion); a sense that one's thoughts were being projected out to others (thought broadcasting), possibly through telepathy; feelings, impulses, or actions imposed by an external agent; and delusional beliefs. Schneider believed that any one of these symptoms in the absence of intoxication, brain injury, or primary affective illness was sufficient to make a diagnosis of schizophrenia. This is not the case today, but questions to a patient involving Schneiderian first-rank symptoms can assist the clinician in teasing out bizarre or hidden perceptual or delusional symptoms that might otherwise go unnoticed.

References

American Psychiatric Association. (2013) *Diagnostic and Statistical Manual of Mental Disorders, Fifth Edition (DSM-5)*. Washington, DC: American Psychiatric Publishing.

Andreasen, N.C., Olsen, S.A., Dennert, J.W. and Smith, M.R. (1982) Ventricular enlargement in schizophrenia: Relationship to positive and negative symptoms. *American Journal of Psychiatry*, 139, 297–302.

Beck, A.T. and Rector, N.A. (2005) Cognitive approaches to schizophrenia: Theory and therapy. *Annual Review of Clinical Psychology*, 1, 577–606.

Dworkin, R.H. and Lenzenweger, M.F. (1984) Symptoms and the genetics of schizophrenia: Implications for diagnosis. *American Journal of Psychiatry*, 141, 1541–1546.

Francis, R. (2019) *On Conquering Schizophrenia: From the Desk of a Therapist and Survivor, with Purview on Metaphysics, Philosophy, and Theology.* Bloomington, IN: iUniverse Press.

Horsfall, J., Cleary, M., Hunt, G.E. and Walter, G. (2009) Psychosocial treatments for people with co-occurring severe mental illnesses and substance use disorders (dual diagnosis): A review of empirical evidence. *Harvard Review of Psychiatry*, 17(1), 24–34.

Hurford, I.M., Kalkstein, S. and Hurford, M.O. (2011) Cognitive rehabilitation in schizophrenia. *Psychiatric Times*, 28(3), March 16. www.psychiatrictimes.com/schizophrenia/cognitive-rehabilitation-schizophrenia.

Martindale, B.V., Bateman, A., Crowe, M. and Margison, F. (2000) Introduction. In: B. Martindale, A. Bateman, M. Crowe and F. Margison (Eds.), *Psychosis: Psychological Approaches and their Effectiveness.* London: Gaskell (Royal College of Psychiatrists), pp. 1–29.

Nuechterlein, K.H. and Dawson, M.E. (1984) Information processing and attentional functioning in the developmental course of schizophrenic disorders. *Schizophrenia Bulletin*, 10, 160–203.

Preston, J. and Johnson, J. (2019) *Clinical Psychopharmacology Made Ridiculously Simple*, 8th ed. Miami, FL: MedMaster, Inc.

Preston, J.D., O'Neal, J.H. and Talaga, M.C. (2017) *Handbook of Clinical Psychopharmacology for Therapists*, 8th ed. Oakland, CA: New Harbinger Publications, Inc.

Sadock, B.J., Sadock, V.A. and Ruiz, P. (Eds.) (2009a) *Kaplan & Sadock's Comprehensive Textbook of Psychiatry*, 9th ed., vol. 1. Philadelphia, PA: Lippincott Williams & Wilkins.

Sadock, B.J., Sadock, V.A. and Ruiz, P. (Eds.) (2009b) *Kaplan & Sadock's Comprehensive Textbook of Psychiatry*, 9th ed., vol. 2. Philadelphia, PA: Lippincott Williams & Wilkins.

Solano, J.J.R., and De Chavez, M.G. (2000) Premorbid personality disorders in schizophrenia. *Schizophrenia Research*, 44, 137–144.

Stone, W.N. (1996) *Group Psychotherapy for People with Chronic Mental Illness.* New York: Guilford Press.

Vinogradov, S. (2019) Cognitive training for neural system dysfunction in psychotic disorders. *Psychiatric Times*, 36(3), March 29. www.psychiatrictimes.com/special-reports/cognitive-training-neural-system-dysfunction-psychotic-disorders.

World Health Organization. (1992) *The ICD-10 Classification of Mental and Behavioural Disorders: Clinical Descriptions and Diagnostic Guidelines.* Geneva: World Health Organization.

2 Historical and Clinical Issues

Introduction

People with psychosis have been treated in therapy groups since the beginning of the last century. However, the approaches have varied, in part depending on the therapeutic theory and techniques popular at the time. In addition, psychoactive medications of the kinds used today didn't come into prominent clinical use until the late 1950s. Consequently, for some 30 years before then, therapy groups were paired with a number of biological treatments, varying from water therapy to insulin coma and electroconvulsive therapy to barbiturates and other sedating medications.

The following sections will summarize issues related to group therapy with psychotic patients from an historical perspective. Trends in technique have moved from psychoeducational to psychoanalytic to interpersonal to cognitive-behavioral over the last 100 years, although various combinations of these approaches also have been used. All of these treatment models have been useful in one way or another, and all have empirical support (see Chapter 3). The group therapy treatment model that will be used in this book takes an integrative perspective that synthesizes the best of these four approaches in an attempt to deal with the pertinent elements of psychosis, as outlined in the previous chapter. Although empirically derived (as will be described in Chapter 6), it was informed by the clinical issues that were pioneered in the past.

The Role of Insight

But before discussing the four approaches, it is important to consider the differing definitions of the term *insight*. Generally speaking, this term for the psychoanalytic (and psychodynamic) and interpersonal schools historically has referred to gaining an understanding of unconscious processes as causal mechanisms for the symptoms of one's psychiatric disorder.

The idea is that by exposing such processes, they can be dealt with in a more conscious manner, thus defusing the underlying affect and reducing symptoms. However, for many psychotic patients, exposing such warded-off and affect-laden conflicts and arrests in development can cause regression and increased psychotic symptoms.

In contrast, insight as used by the psychoeducational and cognitive-behavioral schools deals with understanding the course and vicissitudes of one's mental health problems using a learning paradigm. Troubling psychological conflicts rarely are interpreted, or if they are, their revelations are titrated in small amounts with a great deal of support.

In his book, social worker Robert Francis (2019) feels that this type of insight has been very useful in helping him understand his schizophrenic disorder:

> I assert that insight is my paramount protective factor in managing my thought disorder. Insight is the accumulated knowledge over time concerning the totality of my mental illness...I dare say without insight into my illness, I would be persistently psychotic, highly erratic, and mostly miserable.
>
> (Francis, 2019, p. 63)

As a result of this improved insight, he has learned to control his behaviors despite the continuance of his symptoms:

> Due to improved insight, I may have the same thought content as yesteryear but now with different behaviors. This is the power of insight. Now, when I am psychotic, I self-monitor myself to remain as rational, logical, normative, and unobtrusive as possible.
>
> (Francis, 2019, p. 67)

It should be stated that many modern psychodynamic and interpersonal therapists also speak about this kind of insight when dealing with psychotic patients.

Many people with psychosis, especially during the initial phase of their illness, lack appropriate insight, a condition called anosognosia. Medically, this condition has been defined as "an inability or refusal to recognize a defect or disorder that is clinically evident" (Merriam-Webster Medical Dictionary, 2019). Francis feels that if this condition persists, the outcome for a psychotic patient is grave:

> Anosognosia is used to describe the phenomenon of a prevailing lack of insight. Some individuals suffer madness with no self-awareness into their own irrationalities or of their distinct disconnect from the greater reality...The best outcomes for those with anosognosia are characteristically deleterious. Much of the care revolves around harm reduction, safety considerations, and eliminating any undue emotional distress.
>
> (Francis, 209, p. 84)

Thus, therapeutic techniques that help patients understand the characteristics and course of their disorder and learn ways to cope better with its symptomatology are to be encouraged in therapy groups for psychotic patients.

Psychoeducational Approaches

The main focus of psychoeducational groups is to provide information about the nature and course of specific illnesses (Stone, 1996). The importance of psychoeducation for psychotic patients has been described by Francis in his own rehabilitation:

> The treatment of mental illness goes well beyond simply administering medication...I consider **"psychoeducation"** paramount in the treatment process...Being informed about the symptoms of one's mental illness is conducive to enhanced coping and can be contributory to the overall recovery process.
>
> (Francis, 2019, p. 57)

Although psychoeducational approaches typically use a didactic/discussion format, formal lectures, films, literature assignments, and in-group exercises also may be offered. Patients often are given homework to perform between the sessions. Although the biological and psychosocial nature of the disease using a medical model is emphasized, advice for getting along with others also may be included. In most psychoeducational groups, patients are encouraged to ask questions and discuss the implications of what is being taught with the leader and with each other.

Schizophrenic patients have been treated in psychoeducational therapy groups since the early 1920s, when Edward W. Lazell in a psychiatric hospital in Washington D.C. first described a model that utilized a lecture format and group discussion for patients with dementia praecox, as schizophrenia then was called (Lazell, 1921). He believed that treatment should include educating patients about the characteristics of their illness, informing them about basic psychic development, directing their instinctive demands into more regulated channels, and helping them interact better with other people and with society. Although he was influenced by psychoanalytic theory, which held that psychosis was related to maladaptive early life experiences, his treatment approach was more psychoeducational. For example, he used formal lectures to present issues related to the causes and effects of such topics as hallucinations, delusions, self-love, sexual issues, feelings of inferiority, and the fear of death. During the sessions, patients were encouraged to discuss each topic and interact with him and each other, which added a group therapeutic component to his sessions. Lazell believed that through his group method, patients became more socialized, learned to trust the therapist, and could relate better to the topic areas. This likely was helped by the fact that he preferred a homogeneous format, where the patients who were selected for his group had similar problems. As a result, he believed that they interacted more with each other not only during but also after the sessions, and this helped to counter the negative effects of institutionalization. Although a few patients had relapses due to being confronted with highly charged material, in the long run, Lazell believed that his method was constructive.

Another pioneer in this area was L. Cody Marsh (1933). In his program at Worcester State Hospital in Massachusetts, psychotic patients attended lectures and participated in a variety of therapeutic group activities, such as talks on music and current events, occupational therapy, and discussion-oriented group therapy that centered around their need for hospitalization and the symptoms and signs of their illness. Role-playing, problem-solving, and homework also were included. In addition, there were group activities for the staff and students, the relatives of the patients, and the community at large. The goals were to help patients increase knowledge about their mental illness, including signs of relapse, enhance their coping skills, and comply better with treatment. He believed that "mental patients are susceptible to the group approach" and that "physicians who study psychiatry should have a wide social training and be able to handle patients in groups" (Marsh, 1933, p. 415).

In the 1950s, Klapman (1950, 1951) described a didactic group approach that involved lectures about patient problem areas and homework assignments between the group sessions. He also advocated the use of a textbook, which in addition to its educational advantages also served to stimulate the production and abreaction of deep material during the group sessions. He encouraged patients to discuss the material but allowed them to digress into other topic areas that he deemed useful. He reported that patients who participated in three months of his group showed improvements on the Bell Adjustment Inventory and the Rorschach projective test (Klapman, 1951).

Psychoeducational group approaches for psychotic patients continue to be used today, but rather than focusing on psychoanalytic theory, they tend to focus on modern concepts of the disorder, identifying its symptoms (such as hallucinations and delusions) and coping strategies, relapse prevention, and side effects of medications typically used in treatment (Peters and Kanas, 2014). In their psychoeducational study designed for schizophrenic patients, Ascher-Svanum and Whitesel (1999) included the following didactic topics related to schizophrenia: diagnosis, prevalence, course, causes, prognosis, medication management, nonmedical treatments, stress factors, community resources, substance abuse, and legal issues. In their approach, a lecture format typically is used, complete with blackboard or whiteboard or even PowerPoint, and often homework assignments are given. There usually is an agenda, with the topic of the session laid out in advance, sometimes in a treatment manual that patients have access to. What makes such groups therapy groups is that the leader encourages discussion among the members around key points and then asks them to verbalize how they personally are affected by the issue being discussed and share ways they have dealt with the problem. In one similar approach, psychoeducational sessions were alternated with supportive psychotherapy sessions, with good results (Nightingale and McQueeney, 1996).

Psychoeducational techniques also have been applied in a multi-family group format for schizophrenic patients and their families by McFarlane (2000). Starting with the premise that schizophrenia is a brain disorder that is only partially remediated by medications, his approach attempts to convey information about the illness and its positive and negative symptoms. Family members are taught ways to best help their affected member. Groups typically have a membership of four to eight families who meet with two clinicians every two weeks for up to two years or more. Stuart and Schlosser (2009) also have discussed a multi-family group treatment for schizophrenia that uses psychoeducational and behavioral techniques in four stages: building rapport and alliance, educating families about schizophrenia, using problem-solving ideas to prevent relapse, and applying vocational and social skills training. The approach resulted in a reduction of subsequent inpatient use relative to a sample of patients not receiving the multi-family approach. Dyck and colleagues (2002) reported a decrease in hospitalization rate in schizophrenia spectrum patients who received psychoeducational multi-family group therapy as compared with similar patients not receiving this treatment.

Ivezic (2019) has developed a psychoeducational group model that he believes helps to reduce self-stigma, a common problem in psychotic patients, whereby they internalize stigmatizing views (e.g., dangerousness, incompetence) that are widely held by the general public. Rather than providing a series of lectures, Ivezic's group model uses a discussion format that incorporates elements of skill-building, psychotherapeutic understanding of the meaning of symptoms, working through emotional responses, learning strategies of coping with stress, and exploring different attitudes about the disease. In the process, many topics are discussed, including ways to deal with symptoms, information on causality, the use of other treatment approaches, coping with stress and anxiety, enhancing self-esteem, and dealing with self-stigma.

Psychoanalytic/Psychodynamic Approaches

Psychoanalytic Theory of Psychosis

The aim of classical Freudian psychoanalysis is to probe for unconscious conflicts that produce symptoms, to make the patient aware of these conflicts so that he or she can release anxiety and other strong emotions through insight and catharsis, and to help him or her explore more adaptive ways of dealing with the issues related to the conflicts. Techniques for exposing early childhood conflicts and blocks in normal psychological and sexual development include free association, dream analysis, and transference interpretations.

McGorry (2000) has pointed out that in the early 1900s, psychoanalysts were pessimistic about treating patients with dementia praecox (as schizophrenia then was called) in psychoanalytic psychotherapy, and even Freud believed that they were unable to form an adequate therapeutic relationship. But in the 1930s, Harry Stack Sullivan described a modified psychoanalytic approach that focused on the social and interpersonal environment, both in therapy and on the psychiatric unit, that he felt was curative in treating schizophrenic patients (Sullivan, 1931). As a result of his and others' work, schizophrenia began to be viewed as resulting from inappropriate childhood interpersonal experiences, primarily involving the parents. As a result, a personality structure emerged that was fragile and poorly adapted to life experiences. Even minor frustrations in life produced intolerable psychic anxiety or *Angst* as the psychotic individual attempted to split off and project toxic aspects of the self and object world to gain some relief (Caparros, 1999; Resnik, 1999). At times, this personality structure fractured, leading to complete breaks with reality and the kinds of symptoms associated with the psychotic state, such as hallucinations and delusions. These symptoms and projections of part-objects sometimes produced fear and anger in other people, which led to further interpersonal disruption.

Such factors would be expected to affect patients and even the therapist in group therapy (Lefevre, 1999). If treatment is too aggressive and produces anxiety, this can cause further regression and more psychosis. Therapists should be supportive and create a therapeutic environment that is corrective of the conditions originally leading to the problem. As Della Badia states: "Group psychotherapy is an attempt to repair the damage resulting from faulty early relationships by the containment and detoxification of primitive defenses which leads to ultimate improvement in the ability to relate to others" (Della Badia, 1999, p. 306). Although most modern psychoanalysts are mindful of genetic and constitutional traits making a person vulnerable to early familial stressors leading to psychosis, as well as the positive role of antipsychotic medications, they feel that with support, their approach still can help the patients understand and deal with the vicissitudes of life.

Ego Functions and Schizophrenia

Classical psychoanalytic theory discusses a tri-partite structure of personality. The id pertains to the primitive instinctual drives that propel us.

The superego is the incorporation of parental/societal moral values into our thinking as we develop. The ego mediates among conflicting pressures from the id and superego and creates compromises in our actions that consider the realities of the outside world (Freud, 1926). Although all three parts of our personality have unconscious components, it is the ego that is the most rooted in conscious experience. Ego psychologists have discussed a number of aspects of the ego that they term ego functions. For example, our ability to modulate feelings without being overwhelmed (affect regulation) and our ability to manage libidinal wishes and delay their discharge until an appropriate time (impulse control) are two such ego functions.

A pioneer in the area of ego functions as they pertained to schizophrenia was New York psychoanalyst Leopold Bellak (Bellak, 1949; Bellak, Hurvich and Gediman, 1973; Bellak et al., 1970). He constructed a multi-factor conceptualization of this disorder that focused on the ego. He reviewed over 3,500 papers on schizophrenia and concluded that it was a syndrome with a few common symptoms and signs but many different etiologies and even more different therapies (Bellak, 1949). Concerning the etiologies, he believed that both psychogenic and somatic factors played a role, and he said that "it may be helpful to conceive of any given case as actually occurring on some point of a continuum from a hypothetical point of almost complete psychogenicity to a hypothetical point of almost complete organicity" (Bellak, 1949, p. 740). Note the term "hypothetical." He believed that in all cases, some degree of both psychological and somatic elements was involved. He believed that these causal factors acted to weaken the ego, impairing its ability to control and mediate between id, superego, and reality inputs. The disintegration of the ego produced strange new phenomena (e.g., hallucinations, delusions) and an inability to cope with reality, leading to panic and secondary anxiety that further exacerbated the breakdown. Psychotherapy should focus on decreasing this anxiety, helping the patient to understand the impulses behind the psychotic manifestations, to learn ways of testing reality, and to decide what is rational and what is not.

Bellak proposed a set of 12 ego functions that he thought were "necessary and sufficient" manifestations of ego strength and weakness, which are listed in Table 2.1 (Bellak, 1970; Bellak et al., 1973). He decided to measure the degree of successful adaptive use of each of these ego functions in patients with the schizophrenic syndrome and to examine the resulting ego function patterns to look for subgroups in the syndrome and to compare the patterns with those of other patients. He and his colleagues studied 100 subjects: 50 schizophrenic patients, 25 neurotic patients, and 25 non-patients (Bellak et al., 1970). Through a two-hour structured clinical interview, a standard set of psychological tests, and a three-hour battery of experimental procedures (basically, cognitive and abstraction tests such as Time Estimation, Benjamin Proverbs, and

Table 2.1 Bellak's 12 ego functions in schizophrenia

Reality testing
Sense of reality
Judgment
Regulation and control of drives, affects, and impulses
Object relations
Thought processes
Adaptive regression in the service of the ego (ARISE)
Defensive functioning
Stimulus barrier
Autonomous functioning
Synthetic-integrative functioning
Mastery-competence

Reaction Time), a set of ego function profiles were produced, whereby the various ego functions could be rated on a 13-point scale from least to greatest adaptation. Overall, the schizophrenic patients showed significantly less success in the adaptive use of all the ego functions as compared with the neurotic patients and the non-patients. There was a stepwise increase in mean scores from schizophrenic to neurotic to "normal" categories for all of the ego functions as well. The ego function profiles could change over time depending on a variety of factors, including stress and psychotherapy. The experimenters showed a number of these profiles, differing with respect to diagnosis and condition. One in particular was from an acutely psychotic patient who had very low scores on Reality Testing, Judgment, and Sense of Reality (which the authors found to cluster together in their separate factor analysis of the data). This patient suffered from hallucinations and delusions, which became a central area of intervention in his psychotherapy. After nine months of treatment, all three scores on these factors improved.

Many ego functions are relevant for the treatment of psychotic patients, but two especially are important in dealing with psychotic symptomatology. One of these is *reality sense*, or the ability to feel or think that a perception or belief may not be congruent with reality or the experiences of other people. As discussed in the previous chapter, distortions in perceptions (e.g., auditory or visual hallucinations) or beliefs (e.g., persecutory or grandiose delusions) are characteristic of psychotic states. If a psychotic person recognizes the unreality of these experiences and the problems they produce, we speak of them as being *ego-dystonic*, and patients often want them to go away or at least decrease in their intensity. If these experiences are not so recognized, they are called *ego-syntonic*. A therapist oriented to ego psychology tries to work with patients with psychotic symptoms that feel ego-syntonic to understand how they interfere in dealing with people or other aspects of day-to-day living (in a sense, making them more ego-dystonic).

People who recognize ego-dystonic experiences in treatment are ready to apply a second important ego function: *reality testing*; that is, actively exploring the reality of a suspected perception or belief. A variety of strategies can be employed: asking trusted friends or family if they are hearing a particular voice, checking out if there is a radio transmitter behind the mirror, understanding the relationship between stressful life events and exacerbations of an unusual perception or false belief, etc. As we shall see later, helping the ego recognize the possible unreality of an experience (reality sense) and taking steps to test this recognition with the hope of decreasing its intensity (reality testing) are important treatment components of not only the ego psychologist but also the group therapist helping his or her patients learn ways of coping with the symptoms of their psychosis.

Attachment Theory

In recent years, another offshoot of traditional psychoanalytic theory has received attention: attachment theory. This approach postulates that infants are not able to modulate their emotional arousal, and affect regulation therefore must be managed with the help of their primary caregiver (such as their mother). Strong emotional bonds develop, and the infant can experience distress and anxiety when separated from the caregiver. The interactions between infant and caregiver become internalized and carried into adulthood, producing relational schemata known as attachment styles. If the caregiver is sensitive in responding to the child and provides safety and security, then a secure attachment style develops. If not, then a number of insecure styles may result.

Many authors have postulated two fundamental dimensions of attachment in adults: anxiety and avoidance. Marmarosh, Markin and Spiegel (2013) defined these as follows: "*Anxiety* corresponds to how fearful a person is about relationships, and *avoidance* corresponds to how a person avoids emotional vulnerability in relationships" (p. 5). From these dimensions, four attachment styles result, which are shown in Table 2.2. Secure people neither avoid intimacy nor fear rejection or abandonment. They are trusting and report caring connections with others. Preoccupied individuals tend to be clingy or needy. They are anxiously hypersensitive to rejection and are preoccupied with fears of being alone. Dismissive-avoidant individuals keep to themselves and do not seek out emotional support. In fact, they often push others away and minimize attachment-based needs. Fearful-avoidant (sometimes called disorganized) individuals alternate between pushing others away (due to fears of rejection) and hyperactively trying to make contact (due to fears of abandonment). They avoid intimacy but long for closeness, which results in inconsistent interpersonal behaviors.

Several people have studied attachment styles in psychosis. Strand, Goulding and Tidefors (2015) posit four insecure attachment styles:

Table 2.2 Attachment styles (according to Marmarosh, Markin and Spiegel, 2013)

	Low avoidance	High avoidance
Low anxiety	Secure	Dismissive-avoidant
High anxiety	Preoccupied	Fearful-avoidant (disorganized)

preoccupied (where the child escalates its expressions of distress to meet its attachment needs), dismissive (where the child's attachment system is deactivated), disorganized (where a chaotic style is adopted), and fearful (where the child views him- or herself as unlovable and others as uncaring). They studied 47 psychotic patients using the Symptom Checklist (SCL-90R) and found no statistically significant associations between a secure attachment style and symptomatology. However, there were notable findings for two insecure styles. Significant positive associations were found between the preoccupied insecure attachment style and global symptomatology, paranoia, and psychoticism and between the fearful insecure attachment style and psychoticism.

Harder (2014) reviewed the literature and concluded that the dismissive type of attachment was most frequent in psychotic people ranging from 48% to 71% (versus 27% in a normative sample). In two studies, the disorganized attachment style frequency was 29%–35%. For the dismissive style, Harder (2014) feels that deactivation of affects and impaired mentalization result in negative symptoms and impaired social functioning, and externalization of affect regulation produces positive symptoms. In the disorganized group, she believes that positive psychotic symptoms result from heightened stress-sensitivity and dissociation.

Wickham, Sitko and Bentall (2015) described the two dimensions that are important in attachment theory as follows: attachment anxiety (associated with the development of a model of the self) and attachment avoidance (associated with a model of others). Depending on the values of these two dimensions, four different attachment styles develop, which are shown in Table 2.3: secure, anxious, avoidant, and fearful. They studied 176 people with a diagnosis of schizophrenia spectrum disorder and 113 healthy controls. In the clinical schizophrenia sample, 25.6% described themselves as using a secure attachment style, compared with 55.4% of the non-clinical healthy sample. In the clinical sample, the investigators found that insecure attachment as defined by the attachment anxiety and avoidance dimensions related significantly to paranoid symptoms, whereas there was no correlation with hallucinatory experiences.

Studies involving attachment and psychosis continue both in theory and treatment. An attachment model of using group psychotherapy has been proposed by Marmarosh, Markin and Spiegel (2013). Although the treatment deals mainly with non-psychotic patients, it has a number of insights

Table 2.3 Attachment styles (according to Wickham, Sitko and Bentall, 2015)

	Positive other-model	*Negative other-model*
Positive self-model	Secure attachment	Avoidant attachment
Negative self-model	Anxious attachment	Fearful attachment

applicable to psychotic people. The approach is research-based and anchored in object relations theory, self-psychology, and the interpersonal group theory and therapy promoted by Yalom and Lesczc (see below).

Psychoanalytic Group Psychotherapeutic Approaches for Psychosis

In the 1930s, psychoanalytic approaches in group psychotherapy came into practice, especially for non-psychotic patients. However, Schilder (1939) treated both neurotic and psychotic patients together in outpatient psychotherapy group sessions that met once or twice a week. He used a number of classical psychoanalytic concepts and techniques, such as free association, dream analysis, and transference interpretations. In an outcome review of 49 patients treated in his group, five were classified as having schizophrenia. Of these, he concluded that three were unchanged, one showed improvement, and one recovered completely.

Semrad (1948) described the use of psychoanalytic techniques at the Boston State Hospital to treat psychotic patients in psychotherapy groups. Catharsis and group unity were seen as helpful therapeutic factors. The therapist was viewed as a catalyst who responded to patient issues and did whatever possible to keep the discussion moving in a free and easy manner. Patient-to-patient advice regarding problem areas was encouraged. He described the group work as including patient introspection, mutual discussion and working through of emotional problems, and focusing on reality issues to improve life in the future.

In a follow-up paper, Standish and Semrad (1951) described their psychotherapy groups as meeting two or three times a week in hourly sessions. Although they sometimes had 15 patients, 10 or 11 were preferable. Four sequential developmental stages were described in the groups: increased cohesion through discussion of mutual distaste for the hospital, anxious expression of psychotic material, working through of emotional problems, and termination issues related to discharge. Although relapses were seen in the group, characterized by hostility, increased defensiveness, regressions, and blocks in the discussion, these were viewed as group resistances to the therapist that had to be worked through. Overall, the group was seen as helpful. In a survey of 165 patients (52% schizophrenic) treated in one of 12 psychotherapy groups, nearly twice as many acute than chronic patients who were treated in group were able to be sent home on a trial visit.

In 1947, psychiatrists at the Brooklyn State Hospital began to treat schizophrenic patients using psychoanalytic principles in both inpatient and outpatient psychotherapy groups (Lawton, 1951; Pinney, 1956). The groups met weekly, usually for 90-minute sessions. The therapists encouraged free associations and occasionally made transference interpretations, but in general, their role was to stimulate the patients to help each other gain insight into deep-seated unconscious conflicts. Topics that were discussed included over-protective parents, feelings of guilt, sexual problems, and emotional dysphoria. Although the groups were seen as useful, some members became dangerously hostile toward one another and needed to be removed from the group, and some paranoid patients incorporated therapist comments into their delusional system.

More recently, Correale and Celli (1998) have described a therapeutic approach that borrows from self-psychology and object relations theory. It focuses on the notion of model-scenes, originally proposed by Lichtenberg, Lachman and Fosshage (1992). A model-scene is a scene imagined by a patient that recalls the emotional content of a maladaptive pattern of relationship with a significant other which the patient repeatedly experiences in his or her subsequent interactions. In chronically psychotic patients, such archaic patterns of interaction are disguised through a variety of primitive processes, such as splitting and projection. But when exposed in the psychotherapy group through a description of the model-scene, the interpersonal pattern can be discussed and worked through with reference to the reactions it produces in the group members. Correale and Celli enumerate several techniques (e.g., thematic amplification, controlled narrative, evaluating group roles), whereby the group psychotherapist can encourage the display of model-scenes in the group.

S.H. Foulkes and Group Analysis

Group analysis, or group analytic therapy, is an approach developed by psychoanalyst S.H. Foulkes, who immigrated to London from Germany in 1933. Although psychoanalytically trained, he also was influenced by Gestalt and social psychology. His approach was developed during and after World War II in response to the appearance of large numbers of veterans with various war-related emotional problems. He subsequently founded the Group Analytic Society in 1952 and the Institute of Group Analysis in 1971.

Foulkes saw groups as basic to human existence and influential throughout one's life in shaping thoughts and behaviors in both conscious and unconscious ways (Foulkes, 1964, 1975a, b; Urlic, 1999). But maladaptive groups can produce maladaptive individuals. He writes: "The disturbed individual is a symptom of a disturbed group. The most simple and elementary example of such a group is the family" (Foulkes, 1975a, p. 60). Furthermore, since the family communicates the value system of the culture and society of which it is a member, these larger groups also become influential in development. Since a person's problems result from maladaptive group experiences, Foulkes viewed the healthy group analytic therapy experience as an excellent way to correct these problems.

In his group analytic approach, he endorsed the Gestalt ideas that the whole is greater than the sum of its parts and that the leader should think in figure/ground terms (Foulkes, 1975a). That is, the group process adds influences (such as feelings of safety, support, belonging, and nurturance) that go beyond the individual interactions and that sometimes an individual is in the therapeutic foreground, with the group-as-a-whole being in the background, and sometimes the group-as-a-whole becomes the focus of the leader's interventions, with the individuals receding into a less prominent role. He states: "...whereas some of the therapeutic elements in psychoanalysis are less prominent in the group than they are in the individual situation, other factors come into operation in the group situation which cannot take place in any other circumstance" (Foulkes, 1975b, p. 170).

For Foulkes, the therapist is a kind of conductor of the group process and attempts to create a healing environment as well as to encourage the members to communicate clearly and compassionately with each other in the here-and-now (i.e., during the group sessions as they are occurring in real time). Early in treatment, a patient might view and relate to the group in a maladaptive manner similar to his or her past experiences. But in a properly conducted analytic therapy group, the patient begins to see and experience group life differently. This healthier group experience can produce positive changes and result in a better integration of the individual with his or her outside social milieu. Foulkes summarizes: "The most powerful factor in bringing about change and the possibility for further and future progress after the group has ended is based on this ego training in action and not so much on the insight and interpretation based on words as such as upon the ongoing corrective interaction with others" (Foulkes, 1975a, p. 63).

Wilfred Bion and His Basic Assumptions

Wilfred Bion was a contemporary of Foulkes and another British psychoanalyst who was interested in examining group-as-a-whole behavior. In 1952, he proposed a theory that although the main purpose of any group of people is to conduct the work that it was organized to do (e.g., auto factory groups make cars, student groups try to learn course material), certain unconscious processes develop that interfere with this work. He called these processes basic assumptions. He described these as follows:

> The first assumption is that the group exists in order to be sustained by a leader on whom it depends for nourishment, material and spiritual, and protection. This mental state I have called the basic assumption

of dependence (D.) and its leader the dependent leader (D.L.). The second basic assumption is that the group has met for purposes of pairing; I have called this mental state the basic assumption of pairing (P.). It is suffused with messianic hopes and its leader (P.L.) can best be described as the unborn genius. The third basic assumption is that the group has met to fight something or to run away from it. It is prepared to do either indifferently. I have called it the fight-flight basic assumption (F.) and its leader (F.L.). Participation in basic assumption mental activity requires no training, experience or mental development. It is instantaneous, inevitable and instinctive.

(Bion, 1952, p. 235)

Bion's basic assumptions also can operate in therapy groups, including those for psychotic patients. The group leader needs to be vigilant about the occurrence of these basic unconscious group processes and their effects on the achievement of treatment goals.

Group Dynamics and Group Stages

These ideas developed by Foulkes and Bion that group forces exist that transcend and affect the interactions of its members are part of a notion called group dynamics. Groups increasingly have been viewed as systems of interconnected elements (e.g., leaders and members), that exist in real time, that have a boundary that defines them (i.e., the group circle) and separates them from the outside, and that want to protect their integrity from disruption, much like cells in the body with their cell membranes (von Bertalanffy, 1968). The elements of this systems theory (see Durkin, 1981) go beyond the scope of this chapter, but they lead to many concepts that are used today, such as the notion that each psychotherapy group develops its own normative behavior and that focusing on the here-and-now interactions of the members can be used as a microcosm of the way they interact with others outside the group.

Another aspect of group dynamics that has received much attention by psychotherapists is the notion of group stages. The idea behind this concept is that any closed group that meets for a period of time goes through a sequence of stages, with new challenges that need to be mastered by the members before they can advance to the next stage. A popular system due to its catchy terminology was described by Tuckman: forming, storming, norming, and performing (Tuckman, 1965). Other group-stage theories have been described as well, with numbers varying from three to nine (Beck, 1981; Beck, Eng and Brusa, 1989; Beck and Lewis, 2000; MacKenzie, 1983, 1990; MacKenzie and Livesley, 1983; Yalom, 1970, 1975; Yalom and Leszcz, 2005).

All of these systems of group stages have common features (Kanas, 2000). In the first few sessions, there is hesitant participation as the group begins to establish its norms and the members interact around common goals in a cohesive manner. The therapist is seen as an expert who gives them guidance and approval. This changes in the second stage, where individual differences are uncovered, and the group members begin to compete and even establish a kind of "pecking order" vis-á-vis each other. The therapist is caught up in this conflict, and fantasies of excluding him or her may be entertained. Several patients may band together to attack and scapegoat a patient who expresses unpopular views, and group dropouts are common during this stage. Things calm down in the next stage, where group cohesion is reestablished as the members learn to tolerate and even appreciate individual differences for the insights they give. Intimate and previously uncomfortable topics may be discussed, and the group accomplishes its main psychotherapeutic work during this long stage. The therapist is reintegrated with the group and is seen as a facilitator to the process. The final stage occurs when the group begins the process of termination. Sometimes old conflicts are activated, especially those involving loss and separation, but these are dealt with quickly due to the new insights that were gained in the previous stage. Goodbyes are said, and the group ends.

Note that most of the above comments involving group dynamics and stages pertain to the results of clinical and research work performed on closed groups composed of patients with neurotic and personality disorders. Most of these issues are relevant to non-psychotic bipolar groups as well (see Chapter 7), but they may not be as relevant to groups of psychotic patients, as will be discussed in Chapters 3 and 6.

Psychodynamic Groups

Treatments with the label of psychoanalytic are given by therapists who are formally trained in psychoanalytic institutes. Most of these are Freudian or Neo-Freudian in orientation, but a few focus on derivative schools of thought, such as Jungian institutes. The training in these institutes is carefully prescribed and regulated, and the practitioners tend to undergo their own intensive analysis under a trained psychoanalyst.

Today, psychodynamically oriented therapy is more commonly practiced than psychoanalysis and is more typically taught in mental health training programs (such as psychiatric residencies and psychological clinical programs). Although grounded in psychoanalytically oriented theory, psychodynamically oriented therapists practice a variant of psychoanalysis that uses some but not all of its therapeutic techniques. For example, traditional psychoanalysts may see patients several times per week; have them recall unconscious conflicts through free association, dream analysis, and transference interpretations while lying on a couch; and the therapist is out of their field of vision. Their psychodynamic brethren, on the other hand, may see patients less often, focus less on dream work, and have them sit upright in a chair facing them.

In group psychotherapy, patients already face the therapist and each other while sitting in chairs arranged in a circle to provide a wide field of view that stimulates interactions. Whether the group is called psychoanalytic or psychodynamic depends on the training of the therapist and his or her adherence to traditional psychoanalytic notions. For example, in formal psychoanalytically oriented groups, the group may be seen to recapitulate the family environment, with the therapist perceived as a parental figure and the other group members as siblings. Transference interpretations are common. Therapy may focus on one patient during a session, and attempts are made to expose unconscious conflicts. Dream interpretation also may be part of the group work. Although many psychoanalysts have reported that people with psychosis report fewer dreams than non-psychotic patients, sleep studies haven't found any differences in REM sleep times between schizophrenic patients and control subjects (Stone, 1996). Koukis (2019) has described a group analytic approach to help psychotic patients reconstruct their ability to report dream material.

In modern psychodynamic groups, pointing out the formal recapitulation of the family in the group may be toned down, and transference interpretations are less common. There is more of a focus on the here-and-now interactions of patients during the sessions and less on reports of the there-and-then historical relationships of the patients outside of the group (Schermer and Pines, 1999). Thus, maladaptive interactions can be observed during the sessions and commented upon by other group members. As these can be seen as a microcosm of a person's general interpersonal interactions, what is learned can be applied outside of the group.

The Group Approach of Walter N. Stone

Psychiatrist Walter N. Stone has developed a psychodynamically oriented approach for treating chronic patients in therapy groups (Stone, 1996). His groups are diagnostically heterogeneous; they include not only schizophrenic and bipolar patients, but also patients with severe personality disorders and substance abuse who are chronically impaired. He defines the theoretical aim of his group model as follows: "A dynamic approach goes beyond transactions and tries to help individuals modify or heal old internal wounds, thereby gaining new capacities, in essence to become unstuck and restart growth" (Stone, 1996, p. viii). Treatment goals are negotiated with the patients, depending on their diagnoses and specific needs. They range from improving relationships to problems with medications to dealing with symptoms.

Stone's group sessions typically last for 45–60 minutes for psychotherapy, plus 15 minutes afterward for medication review and management. Usually 12–18 people are on the roster, with six to nine typically appearing for a session. Although the group meets weekly, patients have different schedules as contracted with the therapist, with some coming weekly, biweekly, or even monthly. For this reason, he refers to his group as a flexibly bound model. Patients are not discouraged from interacting with each other outside of the group sessions, but they are encouraged to reveal and discuss such interactions during the sessions if they are therapeutically meaningful.

The tasks of the therapist include: managing boundaries, helping members bond together, identifying prominent themes, managing affect (especially anger), promoting problem-solving, promoting self-understanding (insight), and handling metaphors. Metaphors are given special attention as being clues to underlying feelings and unconscious material. For example, travel metaphors, such as being on a bus and dealing with unpleasant riders, may be a metaphor for the therapeutic journey and feelings a patient has about his fellow group members (Stone, 1996, p. 109), or even events outside of the group that may be displaced to the travel theme. Psychotic material such as hallucinations or delusions exhibited during the sessions generally are viewed as acting out behavior, and if they are group disruptive, they should be contained, or the patient may be escorted out of the session. Sometimes therapists must confront the group when self-learning is being avoided or resisted, but such confrontations should be couched in supportive and not assaultive or demeaning terms. Comments typically deal with the here-and-now rather than a patient's developmental past (the there-and-then).

New members may be introduced singly or in small subgroups of two or three, depending on the referral frequency. The latter is preferred, since it takes the pressure off of being the only new member in the group. The old patients introduce themselves and their own personal goals, often in a formal go-around, so that everyone is encouraged to speak. At times, the entry of a new patient will cause a temporary regression in the group (e.g., producing anxiety or psychotic material) as the members adjust and learn to trust the new person. In one survey, Stone (1996, p. 148) found that 14% of the members terminated in four or fewer sessions, an additional 33% stopped within a year, and 53% remained in treatment for more than one year.

Group Psychotherapy versus Group Therapy

Up until now, many of the groups I have discussed have used psychological techniques to uncover unconscious conflicts that stem from the past, with the notion of improving the patients' psychic understanding of themselves in order to achieve the goals of resolving current symptoms and improving interpersonal relationships. But there are other ways of achieving these goals, such as using lectures, exercises, and homework (like Lazell, Marsh, and Klapman); addressing group-as-a-whole notions to better understand the group climate (like Foulkes and Bion); or using problem-solving techniques and the interactions of group members in the here-and-now as a microcosm of their interactions outside of the group (like Stone). Consequently, to include some of the latter techniques in a treatment model, it is useful to use the more generic term "group therapy" rather than group psychotherapy to describe the approach. Granted, some group therapy approaches also include psychodynamic principles and techniques, but others go beyond these into interpersonal and cognitive-behavioral realms, as will be discussed below. So, from now on, I will use the more generic term "group therapy" rather than the more restrictive term "group psychotherapy" to describe this form of treatment.

Interpersonal Approaches

Stemming from earlier work (Powdermaker and Frank, 1953), Frank (1955) approached hospitalized inpatients with a primarily interpersonal focus. He believed that the goal of therapy groups should be to supply patients with new interpersonal insights that would help them resolve their problems and see themselves more accurately in relationship to others. In this way, they could practice new ways of behaving that would become strengthened over time. He believed that a primary task of the therapy group is to foster a sense of belongingness among the members, which he termed *group cohesiveness*. The therapist can encourage this by keeping the group on task, facilitating member communications, and encouraging productive interactions. But care must be taken to keep emotions in control when working with psychotic patients, since affective contact that is too intense can produce anxiety. Frank was not in favor of a nondirective group approach that emphasized psychoanalytic insight that could impede progress by creating intolerable anxiety.

The Impact of Irvin Yalom

Today, the interpersonal school of group therapy is best represented by Irvin Yalom, who in 1970, published a book on outpatient group therapy that is a classic in the field (Yalom, 1970), and in 1983 a book on inpatient group therapy (Yalom, 1983). In his outpatient book, the group model deals with nonpsychotic patients with the goals of symptom relief and personality change. Because of the ambitious goals, patients often attend his outpatient groups for a year or more. For Yalom, a critical underlying assumption in group therapy is that "interpersonal interaction within the here-and-now is crucial to effective group therapy. The truly potent therapy group first provides an arena in which clients can interact freely with others, then helps them identify and understand what goes wrong in their interactions, and ultimately enables them to change those maladaptive patterns" (Yalom and Leszcz, 2005, p. xv).

Both psychodynamic and social learning principles are used as well, as group interactions may be linked to past traumatic events and current interpersonal problems outside of the group. Typical sessions based on Yalom's outpatient model include six to ten patients and last for 60–90 minutes on a weekly basis. Patients are free to set the agenda and explore important psychological and interpersonal issues that affect their lives.

Yalom believes that grossly psychotic and/or manic patients should be excluded from his traditional outpatient group therapy approach, although he has proposed an alternative model for inpatients (see below). On the other hand, stable bipolar patients may be included in order to address the interpersonal consequences of their illness. In addition, he cites Kanas (1993) and others in supporting the value of specialized homogeneous group therapy for stable bipolar patients that focuses on psychoeducation about the illness, the importance of pharmacotherapy adherence, and the maintenance of a healthy lifestyle and self-regulation routines (Yalom and Leszcz, 2005, p. 631).

Yalom has developed a Q-sort test that addresses possible therapeutic factors in groups. In his approach, patients who complete a therapy group rank order a number of statements that describe ways groups can be helpful based on their personal group experience. Each statement is linked to a therapeutic factor, and from their rankings, the corresponding therapeutic factors also can be ranked in terms of importance. The number and names of these factors have changed slightly over the years (Yalom, 1970, 1975; Yalom and Leszcz, 2005), and currently, there are 11 factors: instillation of hope, universality, imparting information, altruism, the corrective recapitulation of the primary family group, development of socializing techniques, imitative behavior, interpersonal learning, group cohesiveness, catharsis, and existential factors. The relative importance of these factors depends on the treatment setting, patient composition, and strategies of the group. For example, Cabeza (1999) has reviewed six studies using this approach in different settings (e.g., inpatient, outpatient) with different kinds of patients (e.g., non-psychotic, psychotic, substance abusing). He concluded that psychotic patients valued their groups for being supportive and instilling hope that they would get better. In contrast, patients with higher ego functioning valued their group experience more for gaining better self-understanding as a result of interpersonal learning in the group. In general, patients rated identification with the therapist last in their rankings.

In discussing inpatient groups, Yalom points to two big problems: in most cases, there is a rapid turnover of patients, and there is a great heterogeneity of psychopathology (both in terms of diagnosis and in acuity) in such settings (Yalom, 1983; Yalom and Leszcz, 2005). Given the nearly daily turnover, therapists must consider the life of each unique group to be a single session, and he or she must actively and supportively engage the patients in a therapeutic process that will lead to their wishing to continue group therapy after leaving the hospital. Consequently, inpatient groups should focus on six achievable goals: engaging the patient in the therapeutic process, demonstrating that talking helps, verbalizing their problems, decreasing isolation, helping members be helpful to others in the group, and alleviating hospital-related anxiety.

In inpatient groups of higher-functioning patients who are verbal, motivated to work in therapy, and can remain for the entire session, the group typically lasts 75 minutes and includes 4 to 12 patients. A reasonable structure consists of a brief orientation to the purpose of the group (3–5 minutes); a recitation from each member through a go-around of a personal agenda for the session that is doable and formulated in interpersonal terms (ideally involving another group member) (20–30 minutes); an exploration of the members' agendas in the here-and-now interactions of the group (20–35 minutes); and a final review and summary of the session by the therapist and any observers (10 minutes) and with the patients (10 minutes).

In inpatient groups of lower-functioning patients, which may involve those with psychosis, sessions typically last 45 minutes and include 4 to 7 patients. A reasonable structure consists of a brief orientation (2–5 minutes); brief, nonthreatening, warm-up exercises to reduce anticipatory anxiety, such as walking around one's chair three times or doing head rolls to relax the neck (5–10 minutes); structured exercises aimed at revealing personal information, such as telling a partner about important people in your life, or stating things you wish to change about yourself, or writing down things you like about other group members using events from the here-and-now (20–30 minutes); and a final review and summary of the session (5–10 minutes). Sometimes simply getting patients to interact with each other around the exercises without raising anxiety defines a successful session.

Interpersonal Therapy

Interpersonal therapy (IPT) is a form of treatment adapted for group use that views psychological problems as being due to dysfunctional interpersonal relationships. In fact, other than a brief psychoeducational discussion about the nature, course, and impact of each group member's psychiatric disorder, little specific attention is paid to the disorder during group treatment. Rather, the group is seen as a natural laboratory to expose and correct interpersonal inadequacies in everyone. As one's social functioning and interpersonal competence improve, so the associated disorders (e.g., mood problems, eating behaviors) are believed to improve as well.

Each member's interpersonal difficulties are evaluated beforehand in one or two individual sessions. Treatment goals then are established where these can be corrected over the course of eight to twenty 90-minute group sessions. Clinical techniques include psychoeducation, interpersonal problem-solving, advice, and feedback, which are provided by the active and supportive therapist as well as by the other group members. Transference issues are managed but not explored. Although similar to Yalom's approach, group IPT is briefer, more supportive, and has more limited treatment goals that do not involve far-reaching personality changes (Yalom and Leszcz, 2005).

In both the Yalom and the IPT approaches, there is an assumption made that one's interpersonal behavior observed in the therapy group is a microcosm of his or her interpersonal behavior outside the group. Goldberg and Hoyt (2015) examined this assumption in a process study of 207 students participating in 22 interpersonal process groups. Ratings were made on two interpersonal domains, Dominance and Affiliation, through the course of eight weeks. The investigators found significant agreement on how the members perceived their outside-group interpersonal style with their in-group behavior, as judged by other group members. That is, the members' impression of their own interpersonal style matched well with how others saw them behaving in the group. This study gives support to the social microcosm hypothesis.

Process-Oriented Group Therapy

In recent years, many groups that focus on interpersonal interactions in the here-and-now of the sessions have been referred to as *process groups* in order to distinguish them from more didactic groups using psychoeducation. But is this the best term to use? After conducting an extensive literature review, Brown (2003) defines *group process* as "the here-and-now experience in the group that describes how the group is functioning, the quality or relationships between and among group members and with the leader, the emotional experiences and reactions of the group, and the group's strongest desires and fears" (p. 228). Further, she says that process can be interpreted at both the micro (with a focus on one or two individuals) and the macro (with a focus on the group-as-a-whole) levels. Swiller (2011) defines a process group as a "group that studies its own behavior to enable its members to learn about group dynamics, individual dynamics, and interpersonal communications" (p. 263). Thus, it provides an educational experience for nonpatients to learn more about groups, not a therapeutic experience for patients to get better.

For psychiatric patients, a better term to use to describe a group experience, where the group process is used to help them deal with their symptoms and improve their interpersonal relationships through their discussions, would be to call it *process-oriented group therapy*. That is, the therapist uses forces in the group's interpersonal environment to help each patient resolve his or her intrapsychic and interpersonal problems. This is opposed to using a didactic, lecture-driven approach, whereby patients learn to understand their illness and learn ways to deal with their symptoms using more educational and cognitive methods.

Deering (2014) has described a process-oriented group therapy approach for inpatients. She points out that the decreasing lengths of stay and increasing acuity levels characteristic of inpatient units have led to biases in favor of psychoeducational and cognitive-behavioral treatments. Her approach provides structure, while, at the same time, allowing a theme to emerge in a given session, and it maximizes the interactions between the patients, even acutely disturbed psychotic patients. Like Yalom, her approach focuses on the single session and aims to provide a positive experience that will motivate the group members to join a group after discharge. Patients are encouraged to identify conflicts to work on, discuss immediate precipitants and stressors leading to hospitalization, and only address the past as it relates to present functioning. At the beginning of each session, the therapist listens for a common theme (such as coping with negative symptoms or existential despair over being in the hospital) and then helps the group members explore that theme. Therapists are positive and try to instill hope in the patients. Deering believes that in many psychoeducational and cognitive-behavioral groups using a lecture format, patients are talked to rather than being heard, and as a result, there is little space for them to be seen as individuals. In her process-oriented therapy group, the members sit in a circle and are encouraged to find others with whom to identify. By understanding that they are not alone, they feel more hopeful, less isolated, and as a result, form bonds with each other on the ward outside of the group.

Cognitive-Behavioral Therapy (CBT)

Theoretical Implications

Cognitive-behavioral therapy, or CBT, is "an evidence-based talking therapy that attempts cognitive and behavioral change based on an individualized formulation of a client's personal history, problems, and world views" (Tai and Turkington, 2009, p. 865). It traces its roots back to the work of Aaron T. Beck and his colleagues with patients suffering from depression and anxiety (Beck, Emery and Greenberg, 1985; Beck et al., 1979), although elements of CBT (along with many psychoanalytic elements) can be found in his earlier case study of a delusional chronic schizophrenic patient (Beck, 1952). The focus of CBT on conscious thinking was a direct challenge to the behaviorism of its time and as such was seen as a cognitive revolution, or "second wave." That is, to the traditional stimulus-response paradigm, what happens in between (e.g., cognitions, world views, schemas) was put back into the equation. In fact, it was a person's unique subjective "in between" contingencies that were critical to the equation, in that they influenced subsequent actions and could themselves be influenced by these actions in a kind of feedback loop. Learned contingencies also were influenced by early life experiences and the social environment, and they could result in cognitive distortions and negative styles of thinking. In treatment, these could be examined and reduced or extinguished, leading to healthier behaviors. These general ideas applied to patients with psychosis as well, where the cognitive distortions often resulted in such symptoms as persecutory delusions, beliefs of thought insertion, and alien control (Garety, Fowler and Kuipers, 2000).

CBT necessitated engaging the patient, developing a list of problems, and deciding on clear goals for change. Based on this information, techniques could be used to identify distortions in thinking (Tai and Turkington, 2009; Sarin and Wallin, 2014). Examples during the therapeutic encounter included guided discovery and "Socratic questioning" to encourage the use of evidence and reason to examine beliefs and biases. Between therapy sessions, homework often was assigned, whereby the patient identified further problems, tested the reality of his or her assumptions in the real world, performed "behavioral experiments" to examine the results of a specific action, and practiced healthier behaviors.

The A–B–C Cognitive Model

A major theoretical tenant of the cognitive-behavioral approach that affects treatment is the A–B–C model, which Lecomte, Leclerc and Wykes (2016) say was initially proposed by Albert Ellis. In this model, an Antecedent (A), or causal input, is evaluated and interpreted by a person's *cognitive* Belief system (B), which includes longstanding biases and ways of looking at the world (core beliefs or schemas) that may be biologically or developmentally determined. For example, many depressed people cognitively believe that they are worthless or not lovable and react with despair or compensatory grandiosity to stimuli. Many schizophrenic people, on the other hand, perceive the world as a dangerous place or experience external misattributions of their inner speech as hallucinations, believing that these voices have power over them or know everything about them (Sarin and Wallin, 2014). These biased views of the world may lead to generalizations and jumping to conclusions, with the result that antecedent inputs are not analyzed critically. This affects the nature of the resulting feelings and *behaviors*, or Consequences (C), of the antecedent. Since beliefs involve the way that information is processed, changing the belief system can in turn change the resultant feelings and actions.

In the A–B–C model, there is a general focus on how perceptions of events, not the events themselves, influence one's behaviors and emotions (Lecomte, 2019). In a parallel manner, by changing the consequences in some way, this can alter the belief system in a kind of behavioral feedback loop and lead to the way a person interprets his reality in the future. For example, through repeated depressions, a person may have a negative view of the world (B), and when someone else interacts with him or her (A), it may lead to negative actions (C). If a healer can change the belief system (B) through medications or psychotherapy, then the resulting feelings and actions (C) will be more positive. Similarly, if the resulting feelings or actions are directly altered, perhaps through better social service support or via family therapy, then a person learns to believe that the world is not so bad and develops a more positive belief system (B). So, treatment interventions can be made at the level of beliefs or consequences in addition to the antecedent inputs.

Earlier, I discussed the concepts of reality sense and reality testing, which are rooted in psychoanalytic theory and ego psychology. These are two ego functions that relate to the ego's relationship with reality. Reality sense pertains to processes whereby the ego believes that an experience truly represents reality. If questioned, the ego then can take steps to test whether or not the belief is accurate. From a CBT perspective, reality sense and reality testing can be incorporated theoretically into the A–B–C model. That is, one's cognitive belief (B) that an input (A) is real represents a way of looking at the world that affects future behaviors (C). But when the belief is challenged, say by a therapist or other people, coping behaviors can be implemented to test the belief.

For example, a psychotic patient in a therapy group might be hearing auditory hallucinations (A) saying that his brother is trying to harm him. He believes this (B) and avoids talking with his brother (C). But in a group session, the therapist and other group members challenge the reality of the voices by saying that they don't hear them at the same time that he does, and they cast doubt about the reality of what they are saying. Although he continues to hear the voices, he begins to doubt that impending harm from his brother will occur. Furthermore, the group members suggest that whenever he hears these voices, he asks friends or other family members if they hear the same voices and if they also believe that his brother truly wants to kill him. After doing this, and if enough of these friends and family member cast doubt enough of the time, then the patient gradually begins to change his belief (B) and begins to interact with his brother (C). A number of positive interactions with his brother further weakens the reality of his original belief. Note that he may still hear voices (A), but they gradually lose their influence on him. Something like this actually happened in one of my groups—see Chapter 4, Vignette 4.6.

In the clinical presentation of my integrative model in Chapter 4, the ability to sense reality will continue to be listed as stemming from psychodynamic roots (see Table 4.1). However, despite similar roots, testing reality by developing coping strategies to deal with hallucinations and delusions will be placed in the CBT camp (see Table 4.3). This is a change from my previous book (Kanas, 1996), where such coping was viewed as part of the educational approach; that is, learning ways of dealing better with psychotic symptoms. In the 1996 work, many CBT notions were incorporated with psychoeducation, whereas in the present book, the two are separated out.

The Vulnerability-Stress Model

Another important concept in CBT that affects treatment is the vulnerability-stress model, also known as the stress-vulnerability model (Garety, Fowler and Kuipers, 2000; Turkington, Kingdon and Weiden, 2006). This states that each of us brings to the table a set of neurocognitive, neurophysiological, and genetic predispositions that affect the way we interact with the world and its stressors. These predispositions also affect our belief systems and create biases that are less or more rigid (such as occur in psychotic people). There are minor stressors (e.g., late newspaper delivery) and severe stressors (e.g., death in the family) in the environment that interact with our predispositions. Some people (such as those with physical and genetic loadings toward psychosis) may be more sensitive than others to minor stressors. In addition, such people have limited familial and financial resources that put them in a position to encounter more severe stressors (such as unemployment or homelessness) or perhaps to experience more chaotic family relationships than other people. The interaction between predisposing factors and the environment leads to symptoms, and these may be quite different depending on the person's physiological and genetic makeup. For example, a non-psychotic person may react to a social slur with anger or depression, but a psychotic person may react with a persecutory belief or an auditory hallucination. If untreated, symptoms result that in turn create further stress. These symptoms may be ameliorated through a number of treatment approaches, such as psychotherapy, medications, social support, and occupational/educational therapy.

Cognitive-Behavioral Concepts and Schizophrenia

Beck and Rector (2005) have reviewed theoretical and therapeutic issues related to treating people with schizophrenia from a CBT perspective. They point out that these individuals have neurocognitive deficits as detected from neuroimaging and psychological tests (see Chapter 1). As a result, they may exhibit dysfunctional beliefs (such as delusions), dysfunctional cognitive appraisals (such as hallucinations), and maladaptive behaviors (such as social withdrawal, decreased motivation, and other negative symptoms) as a direct effect or as a secondary effect of trying to preserve their fragile mental resources. The resulting "disorganization disorder" makes them vulnerable not only to extreme but to daily life stressors, and the resultant overreaction and production of corticosteroids activates the dopaminergic system, which contributes to the development of delusions and hallucinations. Insight and reality testing ability are deficient, and they have problems performing in work, school, and interpersonal relationships.

Beck and Rector further believe that delusions are characterized by a number of cognitive problems, such as perceiving danger in the environment as a result of feeling vulnerable, attributing blame to people rather than to situations, holding distorted and idiosyncratic schemas about the world, lumping events into categories, and using biased information processing with a tendency toward jumping to conclusions. Reality testing (or "cognitive insight") is impaired, and these patients have difficulty distancing themselves from their rigid delusional thinking and belief systems in order to examine and change them.

These authors report that auditory hallucinations occur in some 73% of patients with schizophrenia, but they also can occur in the lifetime of 4%–25% of the people in the general population (e.g., under severe stress or when falling asleep or awakening) (Beck and Rector, 2005). In people with psychosis, the voices tend to be more negative, are less responsive to corrective feedback, and are taken at face value, whereas in the general population, people know that hallucinations are not based in reality and take steps to ameliorate them, such as looking around for a source or asking other people if they heard the voice or share the same belief. More rarely, schizophrenic patients experience visual, tactile, olfactory, or gustatory hallucinations. The results from signal detection and functional MRI testing suggest that people prone to auditory hallucinations have a greater sensitivity for involuntary imaging in the auditory domain and that they are externalizing this "internal speech" due to an externalization bias.

CBT Treatment Principles for Psychotic Patients

Garety, Fowler and Kuipers (2000) believe that CBT for psychosis has three aims: to reduce the distress caused by psychotic symptoms, to reduce emotional disturbances, and to help the person better understand psychosis in order to prevent relapse and social disability. They see six stages of treatment: building a therapeutic relationship; learning various cognitive-behavioral coping strategies; understanding the experience and meaning of psychosis; addressing delusions and hallucinations; addressing negative self-evaluations, anxiety, and depression; and managing the risk of relapse and social disability. They cite research supporting the value of individual CBT. But they also note the growing interest in applying cognitive-behavioral approaches using a group therapy format. In this, they are supported by others (Beck and Rector, 2005; Lecomte, 2019; Lecomte, Leclerc and Wykes, 2016).

CBT treatment approaches are active, structured, time-limited (usually around six months), and can be delivered in individual or group format (Beck and Rector, 2005). Typically, issues are explored in therapy, homework is assigned to test new behaviors, and a treatment manual is used that provides a session by session progression of themes and exercises. Since a person's cognitions and beliefs are central to the CBT approach, clinical issues focus on exposing them through lecturing, psychological probing, and encouraging patient self-examination. Patients are asked to test the validity of their beliefs by acquiring evidence that confirms or refutes them. For example, in a psychotic patient, the belief that a box contains a secret transmitter can be tested by opening it and using visual evidence to validate his or her suspicion. Note that this process is similar to the reality sense/reality testing process advocated by ego psychologists. By repeatedly doing this, a delusional person gradually comes to recognize which situations are dangerous and which are part of a maladaptive belief system that needs to be altered and made more flexible to a given situation.

Initially, the goal in treatment is to develop the therapeutic relationship through a climate of openness, trust, and support. The therapist at first engages in empathic listening and nondirective questioning, but soon he or she transitions to more formal probing, whereby symptoms are assessed and reframed in cognitive terms. Treatment goals are developed, and education is provided about the role of personal vulnerability, stressful life events, and their interaction to produce the patient's symptoms (the vulnerability-stress model). The A–B–C model also is presented, with particular emphasis on the patient's belief system (B), including cognitive biases he or she may have that affect consequential behaviors (C), and the role of those behaviors in influencing future causal inputs (A). Treatment targets are presented, which in the case of psychotic people, may include interpreting delusions, ameliorating and changing beliefs about hallucinations, and reducing negative symptoms.

According to Beck and Rector (2005), delusions are dealt with by exposing factors that led to their development and exploring the evidence for their reality. Alternative beliefs are explored during the treatment sessions and in the real world through homework assignments performed between sessions. They advocate non-threatening "peripheral questioning" about distorted beliefs to help the patient begin to doubt them and generate alternative hypotheses that are more reality-based. Another technique is "inference chaining," whereby looking for meaning behind a delusion can lead to the exposure of personal traumas in life that led to their development.

These authors further believe that auditory hallucinations are approached by identifying factors that make them worse (louder or more threatening), such as increased stress from daily hassles or feelings of loneliness from isolation, or better (quieter or less threatening), such as avoiding stressors or engaging in pleasant activities. A diary can be used between sessions to record the quality of the voices and events that exacerbate or ameliorate them. As with delusions, the beliefs espoused by the voices can be explored through reality testing approaches. The distress behind hallucinations can be dealt with by normalizing them and pointing out that such experiences are not uncommon in the general population (e.g., hypnagogic and hypnopompic hallucinations experienced by some people while transitioning into or awakening from sleep, respectively).

   Beck and Rector believe that negative symptoms are treated through exploring the reasons for inactivity, examining the reality of negative expectancies and inferiority beliefs, and assertiveness training. Homework can be assigned aimed as behavioral self-monitoring, activity scheduling and graded task assignments, testing new hobbies, and rating events that give pleasure and mastery. Behavioral techniques for dealing with negative symptoms also have been suggested by Morrison (2009) and include behavioral self-monitoring for avolition, scheduling activities to deal with amotivation, engaging (or reengaging) interest in hobbies to combat anhedonia and enhance a sense of mastery, and social skills training to improve isolation and affective blunting.

   Some people have suggested more direct approaches to modify the cognitive deficits in stable, chronically psychotic patients. Hurford, Kalkstein and Hurford (2011) have pointed out that the cognitive deficits in schizophrenia require cognitive remediation (CR) and compensatory approaches. CR strategies are designed to stimulate the new learning (or relearning) of cognitive tasks, thereby improving the domains of deficit. Early programs used paper and pencil tests, but these days, computer programs are available. Examples mentioned by the authors include improving social cognition in small groups and vocational rehabilitation. Most programs use a form of drill and practice training, mitigated by motivations and rewards. Compensatory approaches help the clients avoid areas of impairment and recruit other cognitive domains that are more intact. Examples include effortless learning, which aims to eliminate errors when new tasks are being learned and breaks them up into small parts that then are overlearned, and cognitive adaptation training, which employs home visits to organize the home environment in order to reduce cognitive burdens and reduce the stress of everyday life. In a similar manner, Vinogradov (2019) has discussed a variety of CR and training strategies that focus on psychological cognitive treatment programs (top–down approach) that impact on real-world issues to make neural system change, or direct neurological training (bottom–up approach) that targets presumed underlying neuropathology. Both approaches utilize available software programs and are delivered during several hourly sessions per week for a total of about 30 hours each.

   According to Turkington and colleagues (Tai and Turkington, 2009; Turkington, Kingdon and Weiden, 2006), key techniques for delivering CBT in schizophrenic patients include: developing a therapeutic alliance based on the patient's perspective (i.e., focusing on the specifics and meaning of his or her subjective experiences regardless of whether or not they are reality-based); helping the patient develop alternative explanations of symptoms based on the vulnerability-stress model; and reducing the impact of positive symptoms. Both the content of thoughts and styles of thinking need to be addressed. Treatment targets "include the jumping to conclusions error and biases in styles of judgment found in individuals with unusual beliefs (delusions) and the biases in attributional styles and attentional processing associated with hallucinations" (Tai and Turkington, 2009, p. 867).

Turkington, Kingdon and Weiden (2006) believe that such techniques help patients actively learn strategies of understanding and coping with their symptoms, unlike purely supportive approaches that tend to be more passive, or biomedical models that focus more on diagnostic labels, medication treatments, and psychoeducation that simply contain symptoms. CBT can include but goes beyond the simple neurocognitive techniques of CR therapy, and it avoids the potential regressions from too much anxiety and lack of structure that may occur during classical psychoanalytic approaches.

Group CBT for Psychotic Patients

Recently, CBT therapists have used groups as a way of reaching more people at a time. But according to Yalom and Leszcz, (2005), "CBT therapists were using groups to increase the efficiency of delivering CBT to individual clients, not to tap the unique benefits inherent in the group..." (p. 513). The focus was on providing psychoeducation and cognitive and behavioral skill training rather than using interpersonal learning, cohesion, or group support to effect changes. Group process and therapeutic factor issues were seen as irrelevant or even counterproductive to the CBT enterprise. However, Yalom and Leszcz believe that this is gradually changing and that more sophisticated CBT therapists are incorporating interpersonal relationships and group process issues into their treatment models.

Yalom and Leszcz cite a number of clinical strategies and techniques in the CBT approach that patients can use and discuss in the group. These include identifying and challenging covert automatic thoughts and biases; monitoring mood and activities; ranking, appraising, and confronting anxiety-producing situations; finding ways to solve everyday problems; learning relaxation techniques (such as progressive muscle relaxation, breathing exercises, and meditation); and acquiring knowledge through psychoeducation. The overall goals are to identify dysfunctional thinking, challenge thoughts and biases that have been incorporated into a person's cognitive patterns, learn ways of restructuring these cognitions, and modify subsequent behaviors.

Saksa and his colleagues (2009) reviewed the literature to determine how outcomes of group CBT differ from outcomes of individually administered CBT among patients with early psychosis. Of seven studies reporting outcome of individual CBT in their sample, two supported the value of the CBT treatment. In contrast, of five studies that examined group CBT for early psychosis, four found this modality to be effective. The authors speculate that the reason for these results is that anxiety related to the illness that impairs the effectiveness of individual CBT may be ameliorated with the aid of the peer-to-peer interactions and identifications that occur in CBT groups.

Typically, group CBT is time-limited and relatively brief, with a duration of 12–24 sessions meeting for one to two hours. CBT sessions usually use a lecture format with blackboard, whiteboard, or PowerPoint. Each session typically has a specific focus, and usually a manual is used with an explanation, set of discussion topics, and exercises for the patients to practice, both during the sessions and as homework assigned between sessions. Agendas are specified in advance. Both cognitive and behavioral skills are taught, and group time is taken to review the members' homework done since the previous session. The group leader encourages discussion among the members around the topics and homework experiences. Therapeutic strategies the leaders use include guided recovery, reality testing, monitoring of symptoms, distraction techniques, schema work, and motivational interviewing (Peters and Kanas, 2014). CBT group therapy is very effective in reducing symptoms in patient with psychosis, including young people who experienced auditory hallucinations during adolescence (Newton et al., 2007).

Johns et al. (2002) used a baseline control design to examine a form of group CBT aimed at treating the negative symptoms of schizophrenia, in particular avolition and apathy. The approach used psychoeducation and handouts aimed at understanding negative symptoms, identified strategies to deal with negative thoughts, and discussed behavioral goals that were employed from week to week as homework. Four patients were seen for 14 weekly sessions plus two follow-up sessions, each lasting 1½–2 hours. Despite the very small sample, significant reductions were noted on measures of avolition and apathy.

An interesting neuropsychological study involving group CBT was conducted by Penades et al. (2002). They reviewed the evidence that schizophrenic patients have decreased activity in the prefrontal area of their brains and that this hypofrontality seems to correlate with severity of negative symptoms. They predicted that a group-oriented cognitive rehabilitation therapy program would improve prefrontal perfusion as measured by single-photon emission computer tomography (SPECT). Eight schizophrenic patients with demonstrated cognitive impairment and persistent negative symptoms underwent 24 group sessions lasting 45–60 minutes each over a 12-week period. The structured sessions included a cognitive differentiation component, aimed at improving their basic attentional and conceptualization skills, and a social perception component, aimed at improving their ability to analyze relevant social information. After completing the group program, the patients showed significant improvement on a number of neuropsychological tests and a measure of negative symptomatology. In undergoing an attention activation task, there were small but significant changes on the SPECT favoring increased blood perfusion and an activation in the prefrontal areas, especially on the right side. These fascinating results suggested that the neuropsychological group treatment program resulted in a reduction of cognitive hypofrontality in these schizophrenic patients (Kanas, 2003).

Using a quasi-experimental design, Veltro et al. (2008) evaluated the effectiveness of an inpatient CBT group during a four-year long study. The group was heterogeneously composed of patients with schizophrenia, major depression, bipolar disorder, and severe personality disorders. A treatment manual was used, and groups were held five days a week in 105-minute sessions. Compared with a pre-group baseline year, rates of readmission were reduced during each of the following four years, significantly so for schizophrenic and bipolar patients.

Earlier, I discussed a psychoeducational group treatment model developed by Ivezic (2019) for dealing with self-stigma. Yanos, Roe and Lysaker (2011) reviewed this subject and estimated that roughly one-third of psychotic patients suffer from this condition, which they called internalized stigma. A number of reviews have pointed out the toxic effects of internalized stigma, which has been found to correlate with higher depression, lower self-esteem, and higher psychiatric symptom severity (Boyd et al., 2014; Livingston and Boyd, 2010).

Yanos et al. developed an interesting group treatment for this condition that adds CBT techniques to psychoeducation. It is called the Narrative Enhancement and Cognitive Therapy approach. In a group format, patients first undergo cognitive restructuring by learning to challenge their inaccurate and maladaptive notions about themselves and their illness and then replacing them with more accurate and adaptive beliefs. They then compose and share new positive narratives about themselves with other group members. According to Yanos et al., this method combines "psychoeducation, to help replace stigmatizing views about mental illness and recovery with empirical findings; cognitive restructuring geared toward teaching skills to challenge negative beliefs about the self; and elements of psychotherapy focused on enhancing one's ability to narrative one's life story" (p. 583). The authors offer a treatment manual, where these goals are accomplished over 20 hourly sessions. They also present a clinical vignette and cite qualitative pilot results suggesting the value of this approach for 17 patients with severe mental illness (including schizophrenia, schizoaffective disorder, and bipolar disorder).

Lecomte and her colleagues (2016, 2019) conducted a literature review that found group CBT to be useful for schizophrenic patients. She describes her group approach as being safe, time-limited, and task-focused. Typically, in the first session, the patients receive a workbook in which they can write notes and peruse the text to see the topics and tasks of future sessions. Topics are presented and discussed in each session, and behavioral tasks are practiced during exercises. Often, homework is assigned between sessions, where the patients can try out these tasks in the real world.

In their guidebook, Lecomte, Leclerc and Wykes (2016) discuss the 24 sessions in their CBT program. The sessions occur weekly or twice a week in the outpatient setting and in a briefer period of time for people during short hospital stays. There are four sections to their program: stress and its effects (sessions 1–6), including a presentation of the vulnerability-stress model; ways to test ideas (hypotheses) about the world (sessions 7–12), including a presentation of the A–B–C model; personal impact of drugs and alcohol (sessions 13–18); and issues related to competence and coping strategies (sessions 19–24). Besides psychotic symptoms, other distressing thoughts and emotions (such as loneliness, depression, or anxiety) are dealt with. In addition to CBT techniques and psychoeducation, Lecomte and her colleagues feel that the therapist should observe and, if necessary, address relevant group dynamic issues at the intrapersonal, interpersonal, and group-as-a-whole levels. Measures of clinical change are described as well as obstacles for treatment and therapist competencies. The complete *Group CBT for Psychosis Workbook* for participants is included in the Appendix of the guidebook.

The "third wave"

Tai and Turkington (2009) have pointed out that over the years, CBT therapists have tried to account for the gap between a person's logical reasoning ability and his or her felt emotions. This is somewhat akin to the difference between the ego functions of reality testing ability and the emotional component of reality sense in ego psychological terms. For example, many psychotic people can rationally understand that they are not likely to be targeted by the Mafia, but they still feel that they are being followed, with resulting distress. This dissonance has led to a treatment shift in some CBT circles from merely challenging the content of negative thoughts and schemas to broadening the focus to include other aspects of schemas, such as interpersonal relationships and emotional regulation. This shift has been termed "the third wave" and includes several approaches.

One approach involves mindfulness-based strategies, such as Mindfulness-Based Stress Reduction (MBSR) and Mindfulness-Based Cognitive Therapy (MBCT). These involve training the mind to disengage from automatic and unhelpful patterns of thinking and feeling. By examining one's thought processes (sometimes called *metacognition*), patients are encouraged to develop different ways of relating to maladaptive thoughts and feelings. Sometimes, techniques adapted from Eastern traditions like yoga and meditation are incorporated into the treatment program. As opposed to traditional CBT, where the focus is on reappraising and modifying thought content, an approach like MBSR brings nonjudgmental awareness to current sensations, thoughts, and emotions. Patients are encouraged to "create distance from negative thoughts by accepting that they are there without engaging in their content" (Wharton and Kanas, 2019, p. 363). For example, rather than fighting and ruminating about his voices, a person with disturbing auditory hallucinations would be trained to engage with them while in a relaxed state and accept them nonjudgmentally, thus reducing their emotional impact.

Mindfulness-based approaches have been applied successfully in the group treatment of anxiety disorders (Wharton and Kanas, 2019). Chadwick, Newman-Taylor and Abba (2005) used this approach with 11 patients with schizophrenia who were assigned to four therapy groups, each lasting for six 90-minute sessions. The patients were taught to focus on their body and their breathing while letting unpleasant experiences (e.g., auditory hallucinations, persecutory thoughts) enter into awareness. They were trained to observe them and then let them go without judgment, clinging, or struggle. There was a significant pre- to post-treatment drop in scores on a standard measure of well-being, problems/symptoms, and general life functioning.

Dannahy et al. (2011) describe an approach they call Person-Based Cognitive Therapy (PBCT) for treating schizophrenic patients in groups that combine traditional CBT using an A–B–C approach with mindfulness. In their uncontrolled study with psychotic patients, the negative thoughts they sought to ameliorate were auditory hallucinations. The investigators assigned 62 patients (55 with schizophrenia or schizoaffective disorder) to participate in one of nine PBCT groups that met for 9–12 weekly 90-minute sessions. The authors concluded that around half of the patients improved on measures of well-being after the group ended or at one-month follow-up, and they reported significant decreases in distress or control from their hallucinations, with medium to large effect sizes (0.52–0.95).

Another approach that trains patients to accept their thoughts and feelings rather than try to control them like traditional CBT is Acceptance and Commitment Therapy (ACT) (Tai and Turkington, 2009). Here again, the focus is on noticing, accepting, and encompassing internal events. In fact, the effect of trying too hard to reduce psychotic symptoms is seen as possibly worsening their impact. ACT includes an analysis of behaviors and identification of a person's personal values, which may enhance psychological flexibility. The approach has been used to help people deal with psychotic experiences through cognitive defusion (i.e., encouraging them to view their beliefs as hypothetical statements rather than facts), acceptance, and engaging in behaviors that have worked before in allowing them to reach valued goals and interests (Pankey and Hayes, 2003).

In a controlled study of individual ACT, 80 inpatients were randomly assigned to four sessions of ACT + TAU (i.e., treatment as usual) versus TAU alone (Bach and Hayes, 2002). During the ACT sessions, patients were taught "to accept unavoidable private events; to identify and focus on actions directed toward valued goals; and to defuse from odd cognition, just noticing thoughts rather than treating them as either true of false" (p. 1129). ACT subjects had a rate of rehospitalization that was significantly lower than that of TAU-alone subjects during a four-month follow-up period. Although they showed significantly higher symptom reporting, their rate of symptom believability was significantly lower. Hopefully, such positive results will be shown to be transferable to ACT provided in a group setting.

Compassionate Mind Training can "be delivered within traditional CBT but with an additional emphasis on increasing awareness of negative self-to-self relating" (Tai and Turkington, 2009, p. 869). It targets shame and self-criticism within an individual, with the goals of helping him or her to become more sensitive to self-needs and distress and to respond toward themselves with compassion and acceptance. Therapeutic techniques include Socratic questioning and a "two-chair technique," where a person's "inner bully" can be confronted. The approach may have value for psychotic people, whose voices promote self-criticism and negative self-to-self relating.

Another third-wave approach mentioned by Tai and Turkington (2009) is the Method of Levels. It departs from traditional CBT by specifying that people do not seek to control their behavior but their perceptual experiences. An attempt is made to match these experiences with subjective internal goals or standards, which are in a hierarchy and are analogous to the schema conceptualized in traditional CBT. The problem arises when the hierarchy of these internal goals is disrupted, resulting in conflicts and distortions. The therapist attempts to identify and make the patient aware of these conflicts in internal goals through a probing of associated background thoughts, images, or other perceptual experiences. Socratic questioning can be used, but other traditional CBT notions (such as formulations, homework assignments, and advice) are not seen as being relevant. In fact, such actions may interfere with metacognitive processing and the experiential linking of cognition, affect, and emotion. It would seem that this approach would be useful for patients with delusions and hallucination, and further work in this area needs to be done.

A final third-wave approach, metacognitive therapy (MCT), focuses on the process of thought, especially aspects characterized by worry, rumination, and thought patterns that suppress positive thinking. Unlike traditional CBT, treatment approaches deal mainly with cognition and very little on behavior. Techniques include attention training, exploration of bias, and skills for dealing with metacognitive beliefs that worrying is necessary, and negative information cannot be changed.

Valmaggia, Bouman and Schuurman (2007) described a case study where eight weeks of individual therapy using metacognitive attention training was used in a male schizophrenic patient with auditory hallucinations. The goal was to correct attentional biases by enhancing the metacognitive control of attention. The treatment focused on auditory attentional exercises that paired non-threatening auditory stimuli (such as the ticking of a wall clock or the sound of a radio) with other stimuli. After learning ways of controlling his stream of attention to more neutral stimuli, the non-threatening auditory stimuli were paired with his auditory hallucinations, and the patient was asked to alternate his attention between the two. In this way, he achieved control over his voices, which resulted in a reduction of their intensity and frequency.

Favrod et al. (2014) randomly assigned 26 schizophrenia spectrum patients to receive a course of eight weekly one-hour sessions of group MCT plus standard care (TAU). Another 26 psychotic patients were assigned only to TAU. The MCT group focused on attributional biases, jumping to conclusions, incorrigibility, negative cognitive schemas, overconfidence in memory errors, and theory of mind. The TAU condition consisted of pharmacological intervention, psychoeducation, and socialization groups. Significant pre-post treatment differences were found favoring the MCT condition on positive symptoms, delusions, and delusion conviction. Similar results were found in a six-month follow-up. The authors believe that the beneficial effects of group MCT were mediated through an amelioration of delusion conviction, a dimension where they believe pharmacological treatment had very little impact.

In an uncontrolled, unrandomized study, Ussorio et al. (2016) examined the effectiveness and feasibility of MCT in young patients (ages 18–35) who were in the early phases of psychosis. The patients were all diagnosed with a schizophrenia spectrum disorder or affective psychosis. To see whether duration of untreated psychosis (DUP) would be an intervening variable, the subjects were divided into two groups based on DUP (median split = 12 months): short DUP condition (n = 28, mean DUP = 9.4 months) and long DUP condition (n = 28; mean DUP = 22 months). All patients received weekly MCT group therapy sessions (specially adapted for young adults) lasting between 45 and 60 minutes for four months. They were assessed at baseline and post-treatment on measures of psychopathology, social functioning, neurocognitive ability, and metacognitive ability. Both the short DUP and long DUP patients showed significant improvement from baseline to post-treatment, with a decrease in positive symptoms and overall general psychopathology; significant improvement in social functioning and networking; and significant improvement on neurocognitive measures of attention, memory, executive functioning, and metacognitive measures related to cognitive insight and the theory of mind. In contrast to the study hypothesis that the short DUP group would show greater improvement, the researchers found no differences post-treatment for the short versus long DUP conditions on psychopathology, social functioning, neurocognitive ability, and metacognitive ability. Although this study had no treatment as usual control group and did not randomize the subjects into the two conditions, the results provide some support for the idea that an adapted version of MCT for young adults may be an effective and feasible group intervention for patients in the early stages of psychosis.

Ochoa et al. (2017) conducted a multicenter randomized trial to assess the efficacy of MCT in 122 schizophrenia spectrum patients with onset of symptoms less than five years prior to enrollment. The participants were randomly assigned to one of two weekly eight-module therapy groups: MCT (experimental condition) or psychoeducation (alternative treatment condition). Information in the psychoeducational intervention did not overlap with MCT topics in areas related to cognitive biases or cognitive restructuring. The subjects were evaluated at baseline, post-treatment, and at six months follow-up on a battery of measures assessing their psychotic symptoms and general functioning as well as their metacognitive ability. On the measures of psychotic symptoms and general functioning, there was significant improvement across time in both treatment conditions. On the measures of metacognitive ability, both treatment groups improved, but there was greater improvement in the MCT group. Specifically, patients in the MCT condition compared to the psychoeducation condition showed greater improvement across time on cognitive insight, jumping to conclusions, and intolerance to frustration. However, 23 general linear models for repeated measures were performed with relatively few statistically positive findings, and there was no attempt to correct the significance levels to account for the possibility of Type I (false positive) errors. Also, there was no treatment as usual control group. Despite these methodological problems, the results from the study suggest that MCT could be an effective group intervention compared to psychoeducation for individuals with recent-onset psychosis in decreasing positive symptoms and improving metacognitive ability.

The effectiveness and efficacy of MCT in treating individuals with psychosis can be especially useful in targeting delusions. Instead of directly challenging these distorted thoughts, educating patients about problematic thinking styles and cognitive biases can help undermine delusional conviction. This "back-door approach" is a gentler method of targeting delusions and might help clinicians better align themselves with patients, especially those with low cognitive insight, while also sowing doubt about the delusion (Hua and Kanas, 2020).

Combined Treatment Approaches

In the discussion of the four major treatment approaches that were presented above (i.e., psychoeducational, psychoanalytic/psychodynamic, interpersonal, and CBT), "pure" forms of each of these were introduced. However, in real clinical work, it is not unusual to combine two or three of these together. Combining treatment approaches for psychotic patients in group therapy is not new. Lazell blended psychoeducational with psychoanalytic principles in his pioneering work with schizophrenic patients in 1921, and I have discussed an integrative group therapeutic method for schizophrenic patients that incorporated techniques from psychodynamic, interpersonal, and psychoeducational schools (Kanas, 1996), which will be expanded upon later in this book.

Daniels (1998) described a group therapy treatment model that she called Interactive-Behavioral Training (IBT). She defined this as a form of social skills training that combined standard CBT techniques (e.g., instruction, modeling, behavioral rehearsal) with group process strategies, with the aim of enhancing member interactions and countering the effects of negative symptoms. She studied 10 schizophrenia spectrum patients who were randomly assigned to receive 16 semi-weekly, 50-minute sessions of IBT and 10 who were placed in a waiting list control condition. The IBT patients showed significant improvement as compared with the controls on one measure of social functioning (the Global Assessment of Functioning) but not on five other social competence measures or a measure of negative symptoms, despite non-significant trends in favor of IBT.

More recently, Cook and colleagues (2014a) have proposed a model of treatment that blends psychoeducation and process-oriented group therapy approaches for psychiatric inpatients. After discussing the realities of many modern inpatient psychiatric units, where patients typically are hospitalized for three to five days and receive at best three to five sessions of group therapy, these authors described a brief Process-Oriented Psychoeducational (POP) group approach. Similar to the inpatient approach of Yalom (1983), it is designed to give the patients a positive experience in each session, learn that talking helps, and inspire them to continue on with group therapy after discharge. The process-orientation encourages the patients to interact, thus reducing isolation and showing them that they can help and be helped by others. The psychoeducational content teaches them about their illness and its warning signs as well as ways to cope with its symptoms and avoid relapse. These process and content principles apply to all patients, so the group can be heterogeneous in terms of diagnoses, yet result in a cohesive and bonding environment. The group is intended to help patients with schizophrenia spectrum disorders, mood disorders (bipolar and depressed), and severe personality disorders (especially borderline). The discussion topics are centered on three areas: symptoms, triggers of the disease, and coping skills.

A typical 60-minute session consists of a brief introduction (2–5 minutes), where the group leader describes the goals of the group; a check-in (5–15 minutes), where in a go-around, the leader asks each patient in turn how they are feeling and what brought them into the hospital and listens for common themes to discuss later in the session; the POP session proper (35–40 minutes), where much of the group work is done by (see below); and the check-out (5–10 minutes), where the symptoms, triggers, and coping skills that were discussed are summarized.

During the POP session proper, the group leader highlights themes that were discussed during the check-in and asks patients to comment. For example, he or she may begin by lecturing on the symptoms that were brought up during the check-in, possibly using a white board to highlight his or her points. Then the leader asks the members to share feelings and advice with each other about the points. When the group discussion sputters, the leader goes back to a lecture format. He or she addresses triggers that produced these symptoms and encourages the patients to discuss these as they pertain to their problems. Finally, coping strategies are presented, with subsequent discussion. For psychotic patients, examples of symptoms include hallucinations, delusions, and decreased activities of daily living. Examples of triggers include interpersonal problems, trauma, disruptive life events, lack of sleep, criticism, and substance abuse. Coping strategies are divided into those that are positive (e.g., seeking social support, proper sleep hygiene, acceptance, healthy boundaries) and those that are negative (withdrawal, substance abuse, denial, wishful thinking).

The POP model thus integrates psychoeducation and process-oriented work. It shares some of the characteristics of my earlier integrative model on group therapy for schizophrenic patients and the updated model to be presented later in this book. The authors acknowledge this in a later article by saying that "it is important to note that Kanas's (1985, 1988, 1993) earlier work with psychotic patients, which included aspects of process and psychoeducation, did contribute to the POP model" (Cook, Dobson and Arechiga, 2014b, p. 248).

References

Ascher-Svanum, H. and Whitesel, J. (1999) A randomized controlled study of two styles of group patient education about schizophrenia. *Psychiatric Services*, 50, 926–930.

Bach, P. and Hayes, S.C. (2002) The use of acceptance and commitment therapy to prevent the rehospitalization of psychotic patients: A randomized controlled trial. *Journal of Consulting and Clinical Psychology*, 70(5), 1129–1139.

Beck, A.P. (1981) Developmental characteristics of the system-forming process. In: J.E. Durkin (Ed.), *Living Groups: Group Psychotherapy and General System Theory*. New York: Brunner/Mazel, pp. 316–332.

Beck, A.P., Eng, A.M. and Brusa, J.A. (1989) The evolution of leadership during group development. *Group*, 13(3–4), 155–164.

Beck, A.P. and Lewis, C.M. (2000) *The Process of Group Psychotherapy: Systems for Analyzing Change*. Washington, DC: American Psychological Association.

Beck, A.T. (1952) Successful outpatient psychotherapy of a chronic schizophrenic with a delusion based on borrowed guilt. *Psychiatry*, 15(3), 305–312.

Beck, A.T., Emery, G. and Greenberg, R.L. (1985) *Anxiety Disorders and Phobias: A Cognitive Perspective*. New York: Basic Books.

Beck, A.T. and Rector, N.A. (2005) Cognitive approaches to schizophrenia: Theory and therapy. *Annual Review of Clinical Psychology*, 1, 577–606.

Beck, A.T., Rush, A.J., Shaw, B.F. and Emery G. (1979) *Cognitive Therapy of Depression*. New York: Guilford Press.

Bellak, L. (1949) A multiple-factor psychosomatic theory of schizophrenia. *Psychiatric Quarterly*, 23, 738–755.

Bellak, L., Hurvich, M., Gediman, H. and Crawford, P.J. (1970) Study of ego functions in the schizophrenic syndrome. *Archives of General Psychiatry*, 23, 326–336.

Bellak, L., Hurvich, M. and Gediman, H.K. (1973) *Ego Functions in Schizophrenics, Neurotics, and Normals: A Systematic Study of Conceptual, Diagnostic, and Therapeutic Aspects*. New York: John Wiley & Sons.

Bion, W.R. (1952) Group dynamics: A re-view. *International Journal of Psychoanalysis*, 33, 235–247.

Boyd, J.E., Adler, E.P., Otilingam, P.G. and Peters, T. (2014) Internalized stigma of mental illness (ISMI) scale: A multinational review. *Comprehensive Psychiatry*, 55, 221–231.

Brown, N.W. (2003) Conceptualizing process. *International Journal of Group Psychotherapy*, 53, 225–244.

Cabeza, I.G. (1999) Therapeutic factors in group psychotherapy for patients diagnosed with psychosis. In: I. Urlic and M.G. de Chavez (Eds.), *Group Therapy for Psychoses*. New York: Routledge, pp. 20–31.

Caparros, N. (1999). Splitting and disavowal in group psychotherapy of psychosis. In: V.L. Schermer and M. Pines (Eds.), *Group Psychotherapy of the Psychoses: Concepts, Interventions and Contexts*. London: Jessica Kingsley Publishers Ltd, pp. 83–96.

Chadwick, P., Newman-Taylor, K. and Abba, N. (2005) Mindfulness groups for people with psychosis. *Behavioural and Cognitive Psychotherapy*, 33, 351–359.

Cook, W.G., Arechiga, A., Dobson, L.A. and Boyd, K. (2014a) Brief heterogeneous inpatient psychotherapy groups: A process-oriented psychoeducational (POP) model. *International Journal of Group Psychotherapy*, 64, 181–206.

Cook, W.G., Dobson, L.A. and Arechiga, A. (2014b) Brief inpatient group programming or therapy? Towards a POP model for the RAPID group: A rejoinder. *International Journal of Group Psychotherapy*, 64, 245–250.

Correale, A. and Celli, A.M. (1998) The model-scene in group psychotherapy with chronic psychotic patients. *International Journal of Group Psychotherapy*, 48, 55–68.

Daniels, L. (1998) A group cognitive-behavioral and process-oriented approach to treating the social impairment and negative symptoms associated with chronic mental illness. *Journal of Psychotherapy Practice and Research*, 7, 167–176.

Dannahy, L., Hayward, M., Strauss, C., Turton, W., Harding, E. and Chadwick, P. (2011) Group person-based cognitive therapy for distressing voices: Pilot data from nine groups. *Journal of Behavior Therapy and Experimental Psychiatry*, 42(1), 111–116.

Deering, C.G. (2014) Process-oriented inpatient groups: Alive and well? *International Journal of Group Psychotherapy*, 64, 165–179.

Della Badia, E. (1999) Supervision of group psychotherapy with chronic psychotic patients. In: V.L. Schermer and M. Pines (Eds.), *Group Psychotherapy of the Psychoses: Concepts, Interventions and Contexts*. London: Jessica Kingsley Publishers Ltd, pp. 301–323.

Durkin, J.E. (1981) *Living Groups: Group Psychotherapy and General System Theory.* New York: Brunner/Mazel.

Dyck, D.G., Hendryx, M.S., Short, R.A., Voss, W.D. and McFarlane, W.R. (2002) Service use among patients with schizophrenia in psychoeducational multiple-family group treatment. *Psychiatric Services*, 53, 749–754.

Favrod, J., Rexhaj, S., Bardy, S., Ferrari, P., Hayoz, C., Moritz, S., Conus, P. and Bonsack, C. (2014) Sustained antipsychotic effect of metacognitive training in psychosis: A randomized-controlled study. *European Psychiatry*, 29, 275–281.

Foulkes, S.H. (1964) *Therapeutic Group Analysis.* London: Karnac Books.

Foulkes, S.H. (1975a) A short outline of the therapeutic processes in group-analytic psychotherapy. *Group Analysis*, 8(1), 60–63.

Foulkes, S.H. (1975b) Some personal observations. *International Journal of Group Psychotherapy*, 25, 169–172.

Francis, R. (2019) *On Conquering Schizophrenia: From the Desk of a Therapist and Survivor, with Purview on Metaphysics, Philosophy, and Theology.* Bloomington, IN: iUniverse Press.

Frank, J.D. (1955) *Group Therapy in the Mental Hospital.* Washington, DC: American Psychiatric Association Mental Health Service.

Freud, S. (1926) *Inhibitions, Symptoms, and Anxieties.* Standard Edition, vol. 20, pp. 75–174.

Garety, P.A., Fowler, D. and Kuipers, E. (2000). Cognitive-behavioural therapy for people with psychosis. In: B. Martindale, A. Bateman, M. Crowe and F. Margison (Eds.), *Psychosis: Psychological Approaches and their Effectiveness.* London: Gaskell (Royal College of Psychiatrists), pp. 30–49.

Goldberg, S.B. and Hoyt, W.T. (2015) Group as social microcosm: Within-group interpersonal style is congruent with outside group relational tendencies. *Psychotherapy*, 52(2), 195–204. doi:10.1037/a0038808.

Harder, S. (2014) Attachment in schizophrenia—Implications for research, prevention, and Treatment. *Schizophrenia Bulletin*, 40(6), 1189–1193.

Hua, J. and Kanas, N. (2020) Metacognitive training for individuals in the early stages of psychosis. *International Journal of Group Psychotherapy*, 70. doi:10.1 080/00207284.2019.1704630. Epub January 27, 2020.

Hurford, I.M., Kalkstein, S. and Hurford, M.O. (2011) Cognitive rehabilitation in schizophrenia. *Psychiatric Times*, 28(3), March 16. www.psychiatrictimes. com/schizophrenia/cognitive-rehabilitation-schizophrenia.

Ivezic, S.S. (2019). Psychoeducation as a specific group psychotherapy intervention for patients with schizophrenia. In: I. Urlic and M.G. de Chavez (Eds.), *Group Therapy for Psychoses.* New York: Routledge, pp. 100–107.

Johns, L.C., Sellwood, W., McGovern, J. and Haddock, G. (2002) Battling boredom: Group cognitive behaviour therapy for negative symptoms of schizophrenia. *Behavioural and Cognitive Psychotherapy*, 30, 341–346.

Kanas, N. (1985) Inpatient and outpatient group therapy for schizophrenic patients. *American Journal of Psychotherapy*, 39(3), 431–439.

Kanas, N. (1988) Therapy groups for schizophrenic patients on acute care units. *Hospital and Community Psychiatry*, 39(5), 546–549.

Kanas, N. (1993) Group psychotherapy with bipolar patients: A review and synthesis. *International Journal of Group Psychotherapy*, 43, 321–333.

Kanas, N. (1996) *Group Therapy for Schizophrenic Patients.* Washington, DC: American Psychiatric Press.

Kanas, N. (2000) Group psychotherapy. In: H.H. Goldman (Ed.), *Review of General Psychiatry,* 5th ed. New York: Lange Medical Books/McGraw-Hill, pp. 483–489.

Kanas, N. (2003) Nontraditional group therapy approaches for patients with schizophrenia. *International Journal of Group Psychotherapy,* 53, 388–392.

Klapman, J.W. (1950) The case for didactic group psychotherapy. *Diseases of the Nervous System,* 11, 35–41.

Klapman, J.W. (1951) Clinical practices of group psychotherapy with psychotics. *International Journal of Group Psychotherapy,* 1, 22–30.

Koukis, A. (2019) The ontology and phenomenology of dreaming in psychosis: A group-analytic approach with a neuropsychological perspective. In: I. Urlic and M.G. de Chavez (Eds.), *Group Therapy for Psychoses.* New York: Routledge, pp. 92–99.

Lawton, J.J. (1951) The expanding horizon of group psychotherapy in schizophrenic convalescence. *International Journal of Group Psychotherapy,* 1, 218–224.

Lazell, E.W. (1921) The group treatment of dementia praecox. *Psychoanalytic Review,* 8, 168–179.

Lecomte, T. (2019) Group cognitive behavioural therapy for people experiencing psychosis. In: I. Urlic and M.G. de Chavez (Eds.), *Group Therapy for Psychoses.* New York: Routledge, pp. 137–145.

Lecomte, T., Leclerc, C. and Wykes, T. (2016) *Group CBT for Psychosis: A Guidebook for Clinicians.* Oxford: Oxford University Press.

Lefevre, D.C. (1999) Psychotherapy training for nurses as part of a group psychotherapy project: The pivotal role of countertransference. In: V.L. Schermer and M. Pines (Eds.), *Group Psychotherapy of the Psychoses: Concepts, Interventions and Contexts.* London: Jessica Kingsley Publishers Ltd, pp. 324–343.

Lichtenberg, J.D., Lachman, F.M. and Fosshage, J.L. (1992) *Self and motivational systems: Toward a theory of psychoanalytic technique.* Hillsdale, NJ: Analytic Press.

Livingston, J.D. and Boyd, J.E. (2010) Correlates and consequences of internalized stigma for people living with mental illness: A systematic review and meta-analysis. *Social Science & Medicine,* 71(12), 2150–2161.

MacKenzie, K.R. (1983) The clinical application of a group climate measure. In: R.R. Dies and K.R. Makenzie (Eds.), *Advances in Group Psychotherapy: Integrating Research and Practice.* New York: International Universities Press, pp. 159–170.

MacKenzie, K.R. (1990) *Introduction to Time-Limited Group Psychotherapy.* Washington, DC: American Psychiatric Press.

MacKenzie, K.R. and Livesley, W.J. (1983) A developmental model for brief group therapy. In: R.R. Dies and K.R. MacKenzie (Eds.), *Advances in Group Psychotherapy: Integrating Research and Practice.* New York: International Universities Press, pp. 101–116.

Marmarosh, C.L., Markin, R.D. and Spiegel, E.B. (2013) *Attachment in Group Psychotherapy.* Washington, DC: American Psychological Association.

Marsh, L.C. (1933) An experiment in the group treatment of patients at the Worcester State Hospital. *Mental Hygiene,* 17, 397–416.

McFarlane, W.R. (2000) Psychoeducational multi-family groups: Adaptations and outcomes. In: B. Martindale, A. Bateman, M. Crowe and F. Margison (Eds.), *Psychosis: Psychological Approaches and their Effectiveness.* London: Gaskell (Royal College of Psychiatrists), pp. 68–95.

McGorry, P. (2000) Psychotherapy and recovery in early psychosis: A core clinical and research challenge. In: B. Martindale, A. Bateman, M. Crowe and F. Margison (Eds.), *Psychosis: Psychological Approaches and Their Effectiveness*. London: Gaskell (Royal College of Psychiatrists), pp. 266–292.

Merriam-Webster Medical Dictionary. (Sourced in 2019). https://www.merriam-webster.com/medical

Morrison, A.K. (2009) Cognitive-behavior therapy for people with schizophrenia. *Psychiatry*, 6(12), 32–39.

Newton, E., Larkin, M., Melhuish, R. and Wykes, T. (2007) More than just a place to talk: Young people's experiences of group psychological therapy as an early intervention for auditory hallucinations. *Psychology and Psychotherapy: Theory, Research and Practice*, 80, 127–149.

Nightingale, L.C. and McQueeney, D.A. (1996) Group therapy for schizophrenia: Combining and expanding the psychoeducational model with supportive psychotherapy. *International Journal of Group Psychotherapy*, 46(4), 517–533.

Ochoa, S., López-Carrilero, R., Barrigón, M.L., Pousa, E., Barajas, A., Lorente-Rovira, E., ... Moritz, S.; Spanish Metacognition Study Group. (2017). Randomized control trial to assess the efficacy of metacognitive training compared with a psycho-educational group in people with a recent-onset of psychosis. *Psychological Medicine*, 47(9), 1–12. doi:10.1017/S0033291716003421.

Pankey, J. and Hayes, S.C. (2003) Acceptance and commitment therapy for psychosis. *International Journal of Psychology and Psychological Therapy*, 3(2), 311–328.

Penades, R., Boget, T., Lomena, F., Mateos, J.J., Catalan, R., Gasto, C. and Salamero, M. (2002) Could the hypofrontality pattern in schizophrenia be modified through neuropsychological rehabilitation? *Acta Psychiatrica Scandinavica*, 105, 202–208.

Peters, T. and Kanas, N. (2014) Cognitive-behavioral group therapy in the acute care inpatient setting. *International Journal of Group Psychotherapy*, 64, 272–276.

Pinney, E.L. (1956) Reactions of outpatient schizophrenics to group psychotherapy. *International Journal of Group Psychotherapy*, 6, 147–151.

Powdermaker, F.B. and Frank, J.D. (1953) *Group Psychotherapy: Studies in Methodology of Research and Therapy*. Cambridge, MA: Harvard University Press.

Resnik, S. (1999) A biography of psychosis: Individuals, groups, and institutions. In: V.L. Schermer and M. Pines (Eds.), *Group Psychotherapy of the Psychoses: Concepts, Interventions and Contexts*. London: Jessica Kingsley Publishers Ltd, pp. 97–126.

Saksa, J.R., Cohen, S.J., Srihari, V.H. and Woods, S.W. (2009) Cognitive behavior therapy for early psychosis: A comprehensive review of individual vs. group treatment studies. *International Journal of Group Psychotherapy*, 59, 357–383.

Sarin, F. and Wallin, L. (2014) Cognitive model and cognitive behavior therapy for schizophrenia: An overview. *Nordic Journal of Psychiatry*, 68(3), 145–153. doi: 10.3109/08039488.2013.789074. Epub May 13, 2013.

Schermer, V.L. and Pines, M. (1999) Introduction: Reality and relationship in 'Psyche's Web.' In: V.L. Schermer and M. Pines (Eds.), *Group Psychotherapy of the Psychoses: Concepts, Interventions and Contexts*. London: Jessica Kingsley Publishers Ltd, pp. 13–42.

Schilder, P. (1939) Results and problems of group psychotherapy in severe neuroses. *Mental Hygiene*, 23, 87–98.

Semrad, E.V. (1948) Psychotherapy of the psychosis in a state hospital. *Diseases of the Nervous System*, 9, 105–111.

Standish, C.T. and Semrad, E.V. (1951) Group psychotherapy with psychotics. *Journal of Psychiatric Social Work*, 20, 143–150.

Stone, W.N. (1996) *Group Psychotherapy for People with Chronic Mental Illness*. New York: Guilford Press.

Strand, J., Goulding, A. and Tidefors, I. (2015) Attachment styles and symptoms in individuals with psychosis. *Nordic Journal of Psychiatry*, 69, 67–72.

Stuart, B.K. and Schlosser, D.A. (2009) Multifamily group treatment for schizophrenia. *International Journal of Group Psychotherapy*, 59, 435–440.

Sullivan, H.S. (1931) The modified psychanalytic treatment of schizophrenia. *American Journal of Psychiatry*, 11, 519–540.

Swiller, H.I. (2011) Process groups. *International Journal of Group Psychotherapy*, 61, 263–273.

Tai, S. and Turkington, D. (2009) The evolution of cognitive-behavior therapy for schizophrenia: Current practice and recent developments. *Schizophrenia Bulletin*, 35(5), 865–873.

Tuckman, B.W. (1965) Developmental sequence in small groups. *Psychological Bulletin*, 63, 384–399.

Turkingon, D., Kingdon, D. and Weiden, P.J. (2006) Cognitive-behavior therapy for schizophrenia. *American Journal of Psychiatry*, 163(3), 365–373.

Urlic, I. (1999) The therapist's role in the group treatment of psychotic patients and outpatients: A Foulkesian perspective. In: V.L. Schermer and M. Pines (Eds.), *Group Psychotherapy of the Psychoses: Concepts, Interventions and Contexts*. London: Jessica Kingsley Publishers Ltd, pp. 148–180.

Ussorio, D., Giusti, L., Wittekind, C.E., Bianchini, V., Malavolta, M., Pollice, R., ... Roncone, R. (2016) Metacognitive training for young subjects (MCT young version) in the early stages of psychosis: Is the duration of untreated psychosis a limiting factor? *Psychology and Psychotherapy: Theory, Research and Practice*, 89, 50–65. doi:10.1111/papt.12059.

Valmaggia, L.R., Bouman, T.K., and Schuurman, L. (2007) Attention training with auditory hallucinations: A case study. *Cognitive and Behavioral Practice*, 14, 127–133.

Vinogradov, S. (2019) Cognitive training for neural system dysfunction in psychotic disorders. *Psychiatric Times*, 36(3), March 29. www.psychiatrictimes.com/special-reports/cognitive-training-neural-system-dysfunction-psychotic-disorders.

Veltro, F., Vendittelli, N., Oricchio, I., Avino, C., Figliolia, G. and Morosini, P. (2008) Effectiveness and efficiency of cognitive-behavioral group therapy for inpatients: 4-year follow-up study. *Journal of Psychiatric Practice*, 14, 281–288.

Von Bertalanffy, L. (1968) *General System Theory*. New York: George Braziller, Inc.

Wharton, E. and Kanas, N. (2019) Mindfulness-based stress reduction for the treatment of anxiety disorders. *International Journal of Group Psychotherapy*, 69, 362–372.

Wickham, S., Sitko, K. and Bentall, R.P. (2015) Insecure attachment is associated with paranoia but not hallucinations in psychotic patients: The mediating role of negative self-esteem. *Psychological Medicine*, 45, 1495–1507.

Yalom, I.D. (1970) *The Theory and Practice of Group Psychotherapy*. New York: Basic Books.

Yalom, I.D. (1975) *The Theory and Practice of Group Psychotherapy,* 2nd ed. New York: Basic Books.

Yalom, I.D. (1983) *Inpatient Group Psychotherapy.* New York: Basic Books.

Yalom, I.D. and Leszcz, M. (2005) *The Theory and Practice of Group Psychotherapy,* 5th ed. New York: Basic Books.

Yanos, P.T., Roe, D. and Lysaker, P.H. (2011) Narrative enhancement and cognitive therapy: A new group-based treatment for internalized stigma among persons with severe mental illness. *International Journal of Group Psychotherapy,* 61, 576–595.

3   Research Issues

Introduction

The research literature on group therapy with patients suffering from psychotic conditions generally has been positive. This chapter will review the findings of these studies. Most are limited to patients with thought disorders (e.g., schizophrenia, schizoaffective disorder, delusional disorder), although an occasional psychotic bipolar or unspecified patient may be included in the study sample. Studies involving non-psychotic bipolar patient groups appear in a few reviews, but these are separated out and summarized in Chapter 7.

In Chapter 2, several uncontrolled studies were described that gave important clinical information on group therapy with psychotic patients. Some controlled studies appeared in the "third wave" section; consequently, most of the controlled studies using cognitive-behavioral therapy (CBT) in this chapter used traditional approaches rather than third-wave approaches. With the exception of a few studies on group process, most of the studies in this chapter are outcome studies that compare the experimental group condition with a contrasting condition. The findings will serve as support and background for some of the elements to be described in my integrative model of treatment in the clinical Chapters 4 and 5. Since my model was empirically derived over the course of over 40 years, the research performed directly on this model will not be presented here but will be summarized in Chapter 6, after the clinical presentations.

It is useful to lump the studies of group therapy for people suffering from psychosis into those that mainly use non-didactic approaches (e.g., psychoanalytic/psychodynamic and interpersonal) and those where didactic approaches are prominent (e.g., psychoeducational and CBT). In part, this is because most CBT approaches contain a fair amount of psychoeducation, and vice versa, and both typically employ a structured format, where a topic is presented by the therapist. In contrast, psychoanalytic/psychodynamic and interpersonal approaches rarely employ a topic-focused structure and tend to be process-oriented therapy groups. In addition, modern psychodynamic groups encourage interpersonal interactions during the sessions, while interpersonally oriented groups stem from a theoretical model that gives some credence to each member's psychological history and conflicts, even if they are examined in interpersonal terms. Where possible, the major orientation of the experimental group will be mentioned, but keep in mind that some overlap may exist.

In the studies cited, the comparison typically is between the active group treatment (e.g., psychoeducational, psychoanalytic/psychodynamic, interpersonal, CBT) and a treatment as usual (TAU) or a waiting list control condition, or a contrasting group condition that is more passive (e.g., watching television, discussing current events, support groups). Studies with combined treatments are mentioned but not included in the tabulated summaries at the end of the sections, although in point of fact, there is some overlap within the non-didactic and didactic categories. Because of these confounds, numbers are to be taken as providing information for relative comparisons between treatment approaches, not as rigid values cast in concrete.

Non-Didactic Approaches

Kanas Review of Psychoanalytical and Interpersonal Group Controlled Studies

To evaluate the effectiveness of group therapy for schizophrenic patients, I conducted a literature review of controlled studies that spanned a period of time from 1950 (the advent of antipsychotic medications) to 1991 (Kanas, 1986, 1996). The studies had to meet the following criteria for inclusion in the review: (1) compare patients in at least one group therapy condition with those in a no-group control condition; (2) indicate that more than half of the patients were schizophrenic or partial out the effects of the group on these patients from the others; (3) include at least one major measure of outcome that statistically evaluated the effectiveness of group therapy; and (4) state the duration of treatment in terms of time or number of sessions. A total of 46 studies were found that met these criteria: 33 inpatient and 13 outpatient. Over this 40-year period of time, the studies varied greatly in methodology, diagnostic criteria, and treatment, although in all cases, concomitant antipsychotic medications were used. Formal meta-analytic techniques could not be used without rejecting some of the studies, given their variability, the subjectivity inherent in selecting the most representative measure to use to represent a given study, and the difficulty in calculating effect sizes in some studies due to incomplete information. Since all the studies met publishable research standards for their time and reported significance levels in the outcome differences of patients in a group therapy versus a no-group control condition, each study was taken as a unit and categorized as to whether it supported the conclusion that group therapy was significantly better than, equal to, or significantly worse than its corresponding control condition.

Table 3.1 Effectiveness of group therapy for schizophrenic patients: number (%) of studies

Comparison	Inpatient	Outpatient	Total
Group therapy significantly better than no-group therapy	22 (67%)	10 (77%)	32 (70%)
No differences between group therapy and no-group therapy	9 (27%)	3 (23%)	12 (26%)
Group therapy significantly worse than no-group therapy	2 (6%)	0 (0%)	2 (4%)
Total	33 (100%)	13 (100%)	46 (100%)

The outcome results are summarized in Table 3.1. Overall, 70% of the studies concluded that the group therapy was significantly better than the no-group condition for schizophrenic patients. In the inpatient sample, 67% supported this conclusion. In terms of treatment duration, therapy groups were superior in 79% of long-term groups (37 or more sessions) as compared with 60% of intermediate-term (18–36 sessions) and 56% of short-term (17 or fewer sessions) groups. These duration differences were not significant from each other.

In the outpatient studies, 77% favored group therapy over the control condition. Therapy groups were found to be at least or more effective than individual therapy in four studies that made this comparison. Despite a wide range in number of sessions (9–220), there was no appreciable difference in outcome between long-term, intermediate-term, and short-term groups. Over half of the groups met for fewer than 37 sessions. Attendance rates were high, sometimes reaching 95% or more in terms of number of possible sessions patients actually attended.

I was interested in comparing the effectiveness of the therapy groups in terms of clinical orientation. In all, 57 therapy groups were evaluated in the 46 studies. The description of these groups was carefully reviewed, and the group was placed into one of three categories. *Insight-oriented groups* had the goal of improving self-understanding through the exploration of developmental and conflict-laden issues. The clinical approach focused on traditional psychoanalytic principles and techniques, such as uncovering unconscious material and making transference interpretations. *Interaction-oriented groups* aimed at improving the patients' abilities to relate better with others. Techniques included discussions of interpersonal problems and solutions and comments on member interactions in the here-and-now of the sessions. *Other/unspecified groups* were those that didn't fit into either of the above two categories, or it was unclear which techniques were used or predominated. Examples included Gestalt, psychoeducational, behavioral, or activity groups.

Table 3.2 shows the effectiveness of the group versus the control condition in terms of these three clinical categories. Overall, 78% of the

Table 3.2 Influence of clinical category on group therapy effectiveness: proportion (%) of groups

Setting	Insight-oriented	Interaction-oriented	Other/unspecified
Inpatient	3/10 (30%)[a]	13/17 (76%)[a]	9/17 (53%)
Outpatient	1/2 (50%)	5/6 (83%)	4/5 (80%)
Total	4/12 (33%)[b]	18/23 (78%)[b]	13/22 (59%)

a Significantly different at $p < .0402$, 2-tailed, Fisher's exact test.
b Significantly different at $p < .0135$, 2-tailed, Fisher's exact test.

interaction-oriented groups were significantly better than the corresponding control condition, versus 33% of the insight-oriented groups and 59% of the other/unspecified groups. More of the interaction-oriented groups were significantly better than their controls than was the case for insight-oriented groups in the inpatient and total group sample using the Fisher's exact test. The same was true in the outpatient group sample, but the comparison was not significant. There was a trend for interaction-oriented groups to be superior to other/unspecified groups, which in turn were better than insight-oriented groups in all three settings. In three of the inpatient studies, the insight-oriented groups produced significantly worse results than either the no-group control or other groups, suggesting that an insight-oriented, uncovering approach could be harmful for psychotic inpatients.

In summary, 70% of the studies concluded that on the various measures of outcome that were used, schizophrenic patients in group therapy did significantly better than their counterparts in the no-group therapy control conditions. Furthermore, group therapy was as effective as or more effective than individual therapy for people with schizophrenia in those outpatient studies that made this comparison. There was a trend for long-term inpatient groups to be more effective than short- or intermediate-term groups. Insight-oriented approaches emphasizing uncovering and traditional psychoanalytic principles were significantly less effective than interaction-oriented approaches that emphasized interpersonal problems and relationship issues, especially in the inpatient setting.

More Recent Studies

Despite the recent dearth of research on non-didactic group approaches for psychotic patients, a few psychodynamically oriented studies have appeared in the literature, typically from countries other than the United States, where research on longer duration therapy is more acceptable. One controlled study using psychoanalytically oriented group therapy with schizophrenic patients was conducted in Stockholm by Wode-Helgodt et al. (1988). Twelve schizophrenic patients (six men and six women) were treated with neuroleptic medications and weekly, 1½-hour psychoanalytically oriented group therapy sessions for two years. Their progress was compared with a matched group of 12 schizophrenic patients who received neuroleptic medications and 15-minute "contact" therapy at one to three month intervals with a psychiatrist. About half of the patients in each condition improved, as measured by the Rorschach test, the Defense Mechanism Test, interviews, a self-evaluation test, and hospitalization rates. There were no significant differences in outcome between the two conditions. Interestingly, there was nothing in the material to suggest that the group patients were made worse by the psychoanalytic method used.

Another controlled study using a psychodynamically oriented supportive group approach with psychotic patients was reported from Greece by Segredou et al. (2016). Using a matched control format, 38 psychotic outpatients received a year of weekly, 90-minute group therapy, and were compared to 38 similar patients who received standard treatment consisting of a monthly visit to a psychiatrist for 15–30 minutes. Half of the group patients also made drawings at the beginning of the sessions and discussed the meaning of their work. The patients all were diagnosed as schizophrenia spectrum, bipolar type I, or major depressive disorder with psychotic symptoms. The group approach followed psychodynamic theory, where the leaders sought to understand intrapsychic conflict and the unconscious mechanisms behind the psychotic symptoms. The group approach was relatively non-directive and supportive, encouraging the patients to free associate but also to interact with each other and to express feelings in the here-and-now. Interpretations were kept to a minimum, and the revelation of unconscious elements was avoided in vulnerable individuals, especially if it included hostile, sexually charged, or negative material. The therapists stayed close to reality and commented on positive elements. In half of the groups, making and discussing drawings formed the basis for the discussions. On a number of outcome measures, attending group therapy resulted in significant improvement as compared to the control condition on a number of parameters: general functioning, positive and negative symptoms, quality of life, hospitalizations, and relapses. Psychopathological elements in the drawings also were reduced.

Restek-Petrović et al. (2016) examined the group process in 30 Croatian outpatients diagnosed with psychotic disorders (nearly all schizophrenia spectrum) who participated in four long-term psychodynamic psychotherapy groups over the course of two years. They used the short form of MacKenzie's Group Climate Questionnaire (GCQ-S) (MacKenzie, 1983, 1990; MacKenzie and Livesley, 1983) to see if their groups went through the same group stages that are observed in groups of non-psychotic patients according to the MacKenzie system: engagement, differentiation, individualization, intimacy, mutuality, and completion. Using the GCQ-S, each session was evaluated by the therapist in three dimensions: Engagement, Avoidance, and Conflict, and the sequential scores were analyzed for the characteristics of the six group stages. The groups met weekly for 60 minutes, were led by the same experienced therapist, and were adapted for psychotic patients using the group analytic techniques of Foulkes (1964) (see Chapter 2). The group leader was active and supportive, stimulated patient communications, focused on developing interpersonal interactions among the group members, encouraged cohesion, and avoided discussions of unconscious content and conflicts that might produce anxiety. An analysis of the results found different sequential patterns between the four groups but no clear indications of developmental stages. The general impression was that the groups remained in the first developmental phase. The authors believed that this was due to the difficulties and resistances psychotic patients have in establishing social relations.

This lack of group-stage progression also seemed to be echoed in a process study of 22 sessions that spanned the 12th to 27th months of a therapy group for schizophrenic outpatients (Isbell, Thorne and Lawler, 1992). Using the Group Environment Scale, they found that the group was functioning at high mean levels on the Cohesion, Independence, and Self-discovery subscales, but that there were no changes suggestive of group stages over the 22 sessions.

More recently, Caccamo, Capani and Marogna (2019) reported the results of an uncontrolled "naturalistic" study of 73 patients admitted to a psychodynamically oriented day hospital program in Italy with an average length of stay of four months. The patients who were studied scored high on an alexithymia scale. Using ICD-10 criteria, 44.7% were diagnosed as schizophrenic, 42.4% had mood disorders, 10.6% had personality disorders, and 2.4% had anxiety disorders. The study patients participated in two weekly 1½-hour therapy groups. Similar to the Segredou et al. (2016) study reported above, the mediation group included a drawing activity early on to stimulate later-group discussions, which focused on the sharing of emotional experiences. The other group was described follows:

> This type of supportive group therapy is inspired by psychodynamic theory that uses a psychodynamic understanding of psychosis: behind every symptom or pathological behavioral type in each patient, therapists sought to understand intrapsychic conflict, and related unconscious mechanisms. However, toward the patients, the therapist adopted a non-directive approach and encouraged patients to express feelings, especially in the here-and-now. Group process was based on free associations.
>
> (Caccamo, Capani and Marogna, 2019, p. 332)

The results of the study on the self-report measures used showed significant improvement in general symptoms, interpersonal relationships, and several measures of alexithymia. Psychotic patients were found to have more difficulty in describing their feelings versus patients with personality disorders, and schizophrenic patients reported fewer pathological symptoms versus patients with mood disorders. Despite the lack of a control group and the use of possibly biased subjective measures, the authors concluded that the day hospital group treatments that were used helped the patients symbolize and connect their symptoms better to their thoughts and emotions.

Adding the results of the Wode-Helgodt et al. (1988) and Segredou et al. (2016) studies to the Kanas (1986, 1996) sample suggests that 36% (5 of 14) of predominantly insight-oriented therapy groups are significantly better than a no-group control condition. The Kanas sample showed a group/no group advantage of 78% for groups that are mainly interaction-oriented.

Didactic Approaches

This section will review the results from controlled studies evaluating psychoeducational and CBT groups. In most cases, the distinction between these two approaches could be made, but sometimes, an approach could be included as either psychoeducational or CBT, so some overlap is unavoidable.

For example, where does one put the social skills training (SST) advocated by Lieberman (2008) and his colleagues? In many ways, these programs use psychoeducation to convey information, and some therapists put the approach firmly in the psychoeducational camp (Nightingale and McQueeney, 1996). However, SST also involves behavioral practice and, in some cases, cognitive change. In my discussions below, I have chosen to treat SST as part of the CBT school, especially if the training is limited to an hour or two a day for one to three days a week (which is typical of most therapy groups). Nevertheless, the fact that educational techniques are included in both psychoeducation per se as well as CBT is another reason for the non-didactic versus didactic split made in this chapter.

There are a number of didactic group approaches that are really group programs with multiple components that meet for several hours a day and usually for several days a week. Although useful, such approaches are very staff intensive and costly, and they are quite different from the kind of specific therapy groups that are described in this book. Examples include Lieberman's complete social skill training program (Lieberman, 2008); Roder and colleagues' Integrated Psychological Therapy (Roder et al., 2011); and approaches that combine several different components, sometimes on a single day, such as an hour each of psychoeducation, multi-family groups, social skill training, and CBT (Guo et al., 2010). Comparing such intensive and expensive group programs to the specific group therapeutic approaches focused on in this book is like comparing a bucket of fruit to an apple, so the former will not be discussed going forward. However, some studies simply utilize one module from these programs in a time interval that matches a comparison therapy group. For example, a typical Lieberman module is given two to three times per week in a session lasting 1–1½ hours (Wallace et al., 1992). Studies using such briefer modules are included.

Psychoeducational Approaches: Controlled Studies

Ascher-Svanum and Whitesel (1999) reviewed the literature of controlled outcome studies, where patient education was provided to people with schizophrenia. Twelve studies contrasted psychoeducation with a waiting list control condition, and three others used control groups involving placebo activities, which the authors felt better controlled for nonspecific treatment effects. Six studies reported improved compliance or attitudes toward medications, and another six reported better understanding of illness or mental illness. I examined these studies and concluded that 12 supported the value of psychoeducation for psychotic patients.

In the same article, the authors reported on their own inpatient study of 31 patients with schizophrenia and two with schizoaffective disorder who were randomly assigned to one of two conditions: a patient education group using a manualized didactic format that gave information on 15 topics, followed by discussion (n = 16), or a pure discussion group, where the subjects were presented with the same topics but were asked to discuss their subjective experiences without being presented formal information (n = 17). Both groups met for one hour five days a week for three weeks. Topics that were discussed included diagnosis, prevalence, course, causes, prognosis, medication management, nonmedical treatments, stress factors, community resources, substance abuse, and legal issues. Before and after the group interventions, the subjects completed measures of knowledge about schizophrenia, insight into their illness, and cognitions about medication intake. Patients in both conditions improved significantly but similarly in knowledge about schizophrenia, and there were no significant differences between the two groups after the group interventions on any of the outcome measures. The authors concluded that the patients gained the same amount of knowledge about their illness while listening to their peers as they did receiving formal manualized information that included lectures and media aids, such as slides, worksheets, and handouts. So, lumping all of the above-controlled studies together, 12 of 16 were found to support psychoeducation groups for patients with schizophrenia.

Segredou et al. (2011) conducted a review of group therapy studies that involved patients suffering from schizophrenia or bipolar disorder from 1986 to mid-2006. All had at least 20 participants and included a control condition (usually TAU or a waiting list). Most of the studies were outpatient. In the schizophrenia sample, five studies were reported, where the groups used a psychoeducational approach, and all of these studies reported significant improvement in the treatment condition in at least one important parameter (mainly in social skills, self-care, and general coping; less so in positive symptom reduction). Notably, no studies were found that used psychodynamic group therapy.

Combining the findings of the Ascher-Svanum and Whitesel (1999) and Segredou et al. (2011) reviews, and excluding one overlapping study found in both reviews, a total of 16 out of 20 (80%) showed an advantage for predominately psychoeducational groups over a control condition.

CBT Approaches: Controlled Studies

Roberts, Pinkham and Penn (2009) reviewed 13 studies emphasizing group CBT for schizophrenic patients. Over half of the studies examined outpatients. In general, patients improved in positive symptoms such as auditory hallucinations, general functioning, or social anxiety. Of the seven studies that had a control group (with one exception, either TAU or waiting list), four showed a significant advantage in favor of the treatment condition over the control condition, two showed improvements in both the experimental and control conditions (one used a supportive control and one used psychoeducation), and one showed no significant improvement during the treatment period. The authors noted that few studies examined group CBT for negative symptoms, despite some encouraging trends.

As mentioned in the previous section, Segredou et al. (2011) conducted a review of controlled group therapy studies from 1986 to mid-2006 with patients who suffered from schizophrenia and bipolar disorder. In the schizophrenia sample, eight used a CBT approach.

In one case, which overlapped with a study reported by Roberts, Pinkham, and Penn (2009) above, both the experimental and control group improved, but in the other seven studies, the CBT group was superior to the controls.

Lecomte, Leclerc and Wykes (2016) reviewed 14 studies emphasizing group CBT for psychotic patients. It was not clear how many were inpatient versus outpatient. In general, patients improved in positive symptoms, general functioning, and self-esteem. Of the 11 studies that had a control group (generally, TAU), 10 showed a significant advantage for the treatment condition (in one case including negative symptoms) and one showed no significant improvement. Two of the positive studies also were reported by Roberts, Pinkham and Penn (2009).

Combining the findings of the Roberts, Pinkham and Penn (2009) review and the reviews of Segredou et al. (2011) and Lecomte, Leclerc and Wykes (2016), and excluding overlapping studies, 19 out of 23 (83%) showed an advantage for predominately CBT groups over a control condition.

Mention should be made of a complex study by Drury, Birchwood and Cochane (2000). They reported on the results of a five-year follow-up of 40 hospitalized psychotic patients who participated in a randomized control trial for up to six months of a cognitive intervention versus a control condition of recreational therapy and support. The experimental condition included individual and group cognitive therapy, family education and support, and an activity program with life-skills groups. Although nine months post-treatment the CBT program was found to produce better results than the control condition, after the longer follow-up this advantage disappeared, and there were no differences in relapse rate or positive or negative symptoms.

One factor accounting for this difference might have been methodological: in the earlier nine-month study, the raters were not blind to treatment assignment and might have been biased in favor of the CBT condition; in the longer follow-up study, they were blind to treatment. Interestingly, some of the CBT gains persisted in patients that had no or only one relapse in the intervening period, leading the authors to suggest that CBT applied in the acute phase of a psychotic disorder can produce enduring benefit if subsequent relapses can be minimized. They suggest that relapse prevention programs or periodic "booster sessions" might be helpful in the long-term care of these patients.

Meta-Analytic Studies

Four meta-analyses have been conducted on studies that used didactic approaches in group therapy with psychotic patients. Wykes et al. (2008) reviewed 34 studies examining the effects of cognitive behavior therapy on targeted symptoms in psychotic patients (the majority of whom were schizophrenic). All patients received standard psychiatric care including medications (the TAU condition). Patients were randomized to receive CBT versus TAU alone, and in some cases, a control treatment (such as supportive therapy or a placebo such as befriending). Overall, a modest effect size of 0.40 was found in the studies favoring CBT. There were no significant differences in effect size between the seven studies that used group CBT (ES = 0.39) and the remainder that used individual CBT (ES = 0.42). Effect sizes ranging between 0.35 and 0.44 were found for targeted issues that included positive symptoms, negative symptoms, general functioning, mood, and social anxiety; only hopelessness was found to produce a non-significant effect. Trials in which the raters were aware of the group allocation had an inflated effect size of about 50%–100%, showing the influence of treatment allocation bias. Nevertheless, the blind studies still gave an effect size of 0.22.

Xia, Merinder and Belgamwar (2011) conducted a meta-analysis of randomized controlled studies that focused on psychoeducation for schizophrenia and related serious mental illnesses involving individuals or groups. Data were extracted involving 5,142 participants (mostly in-patients) from 44 trials conducted between 1988 and 2009. The median study duration was around 12 weeks. Based on their meta-analysis, the incidences of noncompliance with medication, length of hospital stay, illness relapse, and hospital readmissions were each significantly lower in the psychoeducational condition. Patients in the psychoeducational condition also were more likely to be satisfied with their mental health services, to have improved quality of life, and to exhibit better social and global functioning.

In a third meta-analysis, Orfanos, Banks and Priebe (2014) conduced an evaluation of studies going back several decades from March 2014. Thirty-two studies were found that included a randomized controlled format: 19 data sets compared a group therapeutic treatment to TAU, and 13 data sets compared a group therapeutic treatment to an active sham group. There were a total of 2,634 adult patients, and 85% or more were diagnosed with schizophrenia or a related condition. The group therapy breakdown was: CBT approaches, including social skills or compensatory cognitive training (31%); non-verbal arts therapy, such as music or body-oriented therapy (19%); and others, such as cognitive remediation (CR) therapy and psychoeducation (50%). Seventy-one percent were outpatient studies, and just under two-thirds of the patients were male. There were significant advantages of the therapy groups over the TAU condition in improving negative symptoms but not positive symptoms. The effect size on negative symptoms was moderated by treatment intensity (number of sessions), and narrative summaries suggested that participants in group therapy benefited more in terms of improving social functioning in the group therapy versus TAU condition. Although total and general symptoms also improved, these advantages lost their significance when a sensitivity analysis was made to exclude studies judged to be biased. There were no differences between the therapy and sham groups on any of the measures, nor was there evidence for an effect of therapeutic orientation in the groups that were studied. The authors concluded that non-specific group therapy mechanisms can be useful for schizophrenic patients, especially as regards negative symptoms and social deficits. The authors could not explain the absence of effect on positive symptoms other than to speculate that less heterogeneous groups specializing in one symptom, such as hallucinations or delusions, might be more effective.

Another meta-analysis of studies on group therapy with schizophrenic patients was conducted by Burlingame et al. (2020). The authors searched databases from 1990 to 2018 and found 52 studies of 4,156 individuals that used randomized controlled trials that evaluated the effects of seven group treatments on positive and negative symptoms of schizophrenia. Studies were included if 85% or more of the patients had a schizophrenia spectrum disorder, and the control conditions included TAU (nearly two-thirds of the contrasts), an active control, a waiting list, and medication. Typically, groups had 18 bi-weekly sessions of 75 minutes each. Treatment manuals were used in 78.4% of the groups, but only 36.7% had adherence checks. Overall, there were small effects ($g = 0.30$) favoring the group treatments over controls, and effect sizes for treatment-specific outcomes were higher than those for general outcomes. There were no significant differences between improvements in positive ($g = 0.34$) versus negative ($g = 0.27$) symptoms. Four of the studied treatments resulted in significant effect sizes: CR, the most studied and second most effective treatment; SST, which had the largest effects when contrasted against all other treatment approaches; patient psychoeducation (PE); and multi-family groups. CBT, metacognitive training, and combinations of SST, PE, and CR were not associated with improvements. Group leader training and dose of treatment (number of sessions) improved treatment-specific outcomes.

Other Studies

Lecomte and her colleagues (2008) evaluated the effectiveness of group CBT on 129 patients with recent onset psychosis. They conducted a single-blind, randomized controlled trial, where patients were randomized into one of three conditions: 24 semiweekly sessions of group CBT, SST for symptom management, and a wait-list control. The results at post-therapy and at six-month follow-up revealed that both treatment interventions were superior to the control condition in terms of reducing positive and negative symptoms. Only the CBT patients showed improvement in self-esteem, social support, and the use of active coping strategies in dealing with stress.

Lecomte and her colleagues (2012) did a one-year follow-up on these patients. There was high attrition by the 12-month post-therapy assessment time, especially in the social skills and wait-list conditions, so only patients who completed over half of the CBT groups could be evaluated. Negative symptoms remained low, but positive symptoms returned to nearly pre-therapy levels. There was significant improvement in the group CBT condition for social support and insight. Scores on measures of malevolence and omnipotence in auditory hallucinations decreased.

Lessons Learned

The above-controlled studies of group treatments from various schools of thought support the notion that group therapy as a treatment modality is helpful for psychotic patients. Combining the results from several large reviews, 78% of groups using a predominately interaction-oriented, interpersonal focus were significantly better than their control groups versus 80% of psychoeducational groups and 83% of CBT groups. Only groups focusing on a psychoanalytic, insight-orientation scored lower: 36% of such groups were better than their controls, and in some of these groups, patients performed significantly worse than controls. Many of the insight-oriented group studies were older and used a more traditional psychoanalytic approach than the psychodynamic models that are used today, which include more support and less uncovering (see Segredou et al. (2016). Nevertheless, it appears that approaches that excessively arouse emotions and produce anxiety can aggravate symptoms and cause regression in psychotic patients. More research needs to be done on modern psychodynamic groups with psychotic patients to see which factors can improve their effectiveness without causing harm.

Unfortunately, in the past two decades, there have been relatively few controlled studies of group therapy with psychotic patients using non-didactic as compared with didactic approaches, especially CBT (Burlingame, Strauss and Joyce, 2013; Kanas, 2019; Peters and Kanas, 2014). There are several reasons for this. CBT treatments have specific agendas and measurable outcome goals that are well suited for research, since they tend to be manualized, which allows therapy adherence and outcome to be measured. In contrast, non-didactic approaches tend to be more open-ended, with patients setting the agenda each session in less predictable ways. Also, CBT tends to be time-limited and relatively short-term, whereas psychodynamic and interpersonal therapies tend to be longer with more broad-based goals. All these factors favor the procurement of research funding for CBT, so more studies have been done using this treatment modality. Tost et al. (1999) have pointed out that the flexible and spontaneous nature of non-didactive approaches, as well as their emphasis on subjective and subtle changes in patients undergoing treatment, do not lend themselves to an experimental framework. This is not to say that modern non-didactic group approaches are all ineffective or do not help psychotic patients improve in their symptomatology and interpersonal relationships, but rather, the research using these approaches is just not being done. Hopefully, future investigators will develop proposals meeting current research criteria to test the effectiveness of these non-didactic treatment methods.

Svien and Burlingame (2019) have pointed out that there seems to be a trend in group treatments toward composing groups with specific patient populations and defining specific treatment targets, and groups with psychotic patients are no exception. They state: "Modern groups for persons with schizophrenia typically focus on mitigating specific symptoms in psychotic-spectrum disorders" (p. 351), especially cognitive impairments using didactic approaches. They review the results from two studies in support of this thesis, one targeting cognitive distortions and positive symptoms like auditory hallucinations and delusions (Favrod et al., 2014) and the other targeting seven behaviors involved in social interactions (Rus-Calafell et al., 2013). This trend toward specific treatment goals and outcomes may be influenced by current managed care practices and evidence-based priorities. This likely is another reason why traditional group approaches (such as those involving psychodynamic or interpersonal techniques) that have more global treatment goals are not as prevalent in the recent research literature.

The four approaches mentioned above (psychoanalytical/psychodynamic, interpersonal, psychoeducational, and CBT) focus on different aspects of psychosis which can be helpful for these patients. These range from gaining a better understanding of their disease and its vicissitudes, to learning strategies of coping with their symptoms, to becoming better able to sense and test reality, to experimenting with different cognitive and behavioral strategies, to improving their interpersonal relationships. It would seem that an *integrative* group therapeutic approach that borrows the best from these four schools and produces a safe, supportive environment would be recommended for people suffering from psychotic disorders. It is to such an approach that we now turn.

References

Ascher-Svanum, H. and Whitesel, J. (1999) A randomized controlled study of two styles of group patient education about schizophrenia. *Psychiatric Services*, 50, 926–930.

Burlingame, G.M., Strauss, B. and Joyce, A.S. (2013) Change mechanisms and effectiveness of small group treatments. In: M.J. Lambert (Ed.), *Bergin and Garfield's Handbook of Psychotherapy and Behavior Change,* 6th ed. New York: Wiley and Sons, pp. 640–689.

Burlingame, G.M., Svien, H., Hoppe, L., Hunt, I. and Rosendahl, J. (2020) Group therapy for schizophrenia: A meta-analysis. *Psychotherapy*, 57, 219–236.

Caccamo, F., Capani, A., and Marogna, C. (2019) Evaluation of symptoms and alexithymia in psychiatric patients: A naturalistic longitudinal study in a day hospital. *International Journal of Group Psychotherapy*, 69, 328–344.

Drury, V., Birchwood, M., and Cochrane, R. (2000) Cognitive therapy and recovery from acute psychosis: A controlled trial. 3. Five-year follow-up. *British Journal of Psychiatry*, 177(1), 8–14.

Favrod, J., Rexhaj, S., Bardy, S., Ferrari, P., Hayoz, C., Moritz, S., … Bonsack, C. (2014) Sustained antipsychotic effect of metacognitive training in psychosis: A randomized-controlled study. *European Psychiatry*, 29, 275–281.

Foulkes, S.H. (1964) *Therapeutic Group Analysis*. London: Karnac Books.

Guo, X., Zhai, J., Liu, Z., Fang, M., Wang, B., Wang, C. and Zhao, J. (2010) Effect of antipsychotic medication alone vs. combined with psychosocial intervention on outcomes of early-stage schizophrenia: A randomized, 1-year study. *Archives of General Psychiatry*, 67(9), 895–904.

Isbell, S.E., Thorne, A. and Lawler, M.H. (1992) An exploratory study of videotapes of long-term group psychotherapy of outpatients with major and chronic mental illness. *Group*, 16, 101–111.

Kanas, N. (1986) Group therapy with schizophrenics: A review of controlled studies. *International Journal of Group Psychotherapy*, 36, 339–351.

Kanas, N. (1996) *Group Therapy for Schizophrenic Patients*. Washington, D.C.: American Psychiatric Press.

Kanas, N. (2019) Research review: Editor's note. *International Journal of Group Psychotherapy*, 69, 345–346.

Lecomte, T., Leclerc, C. and Wykes, T. (2012) Group CBT for early psychosis—Are there still benefits one year later? *International Journal of Group Psychotherapy*, 62, 309–321.

Lecomte, T., Leclerc, C. and Wykes, T. (2016) *Group CBT for Psychosis: A Guidebook for Clinicians*. Oxford, UK: Oxford University Press.

Lecomte, T., Leclerc, C., Corbiere, M., Wykes, T., Wallace, C.J. and Spidel, A. (2008) Group cognitive behavior therapy or social skills training for individuals with a recent onset of psychosis?: Results of a randomized controlled trial. *Journal of Nervous and Mental Disease*, 196, 866–875.

Lieberman, R.P. (2008) *Recovery from Disability: Manual of Psychiatric Rehabilitation*. Washington, D.C.: American Psychiatric Press.

MacKenzie, K.R. (1983) The clinical application of a group climate measure. In: R.R. Dies and K.R. Makenzie (Eds.), *Advances in Group Psychotherapy: Integrating Research and Practice*. New York: International Universities Press, pp. 159–170.

MacKenzie, K.R. (1990) *Introduction to Time-Limited Group Psychotherapy*. Washington, D.C.: American Psychiatric Press.

MacKenzie, K.R. and Livesley, W.J. (1983) A developmental model for brief group therapy. In: R.R. Dies and K.R. Makenzie (Eds.), *Advances in Group Psychotherapy: Integrating Research and Practice*. New York: International Universities Press, pp. 101–116.

Nightingale, L.C. and McQueeney, D.A. (1996) Group therapy for schizophrenia: Combining and expanding the psychoeducational model with supportive psychotherapy. *International Journal of Group Psychotherapy*, 46(4), 517–533.

Orfanos, S., Banks, C. and Priebe, S. (2014) Are group psychotherapeutic treatments effective for patients with schizophrenia? A systematic review and meta-analysis. *Psychotherapy and Psychosomatics*, 84, 241–249.

Peters, T. and Kanas, N. (2014) Psychodynamic research in group therapy. *International Journal of Group Psychotherapy*, 64, 587–591.

Restek-Petrović, B., Gregurek, R., Petrović, R., Orešković-Krezler, N., Mihanović, M. and Ivezić, E. (2016) Characteristics of the group process in long-term psychodynamic group psychotherapy for patients with psychosis. *International Journal of Group Psychotherapy*, 66, 132–143.

Roberts, D.L., Pinkham, A.E. and Penn, D.L. (2009) Schizophrenia. In: P.J. Bieling, R.E. McCabe and M.M. Antony (Eds.), *Cognitive-Behavioral Therapy in Groups*. New York: Guilford Press, pp. 350–371.

Roder, V., Müller, D.R., Brenner, H.D. and Spaulding, W.D. (2011) *Integrated Psychological Therapy (IPT) for the Treatment of Neurocognition, Social Cognition, and Social Competency in Schizophrenia Patients*. Cambridge, MA: Hogrefe Publishing.

Rus-Calafell, M., Gutiérrez-Maldonado, J., Ortega-Bravo, M., Ribas-Sabaté, J. and Caqueo-Urízar, A. (2013). A brief cognitive-behavioral social skills training for stabilized outpatients with schizophrenia: A preliminary study. *Schizophrenia Research*, 143, 327–336.

Segredou, I., Christodoulou, C., Samakouri, M., Antoniadou, O., Poulis, E., Therapou, K. and Livaditis, M. (2016) Psychodynamically oriented supportive group therapy with psychotic patients. *Small Group Research*, 47(2), 155–176.

Segredou, I., Xenitidis, K., Panagiotopoulou, M., Bochtsou, V., Antoniadou, O. and Livaditis, M. (2011) Group psychosocial interventions for adults with schizophrenia and bipolar illness: The evidence base in the light of publications between 1986 and 2006. *International Journal of Social Psychiatry*, 58, 229–238.

Svien, H. and Burlingame, G.M. (2019) Trends in modern group psychotherapy for schizophrenia. *International Journal of Group Psychotherapy*, 69, 347–352.

Tost, L., Tost, D., Hernandez, C. and De Chavez, M.G. (1999) Limitations of nomothetic procedures for group psychotherapy in psychosis. In: I. Urlic and M.G. de Chavez (Eds.), *Group Therapy for Psychoses*. New York: Routledge, pp. 11–19.

Wallace, C.J., Liberman, R.P., MacKain, S.J., Blackwell, G. and Eckman, T.A. (1992) Effectiveness and replicability of modules for teaching social and instrumental skills to the severely mentally ill. *American Journal of Psychiatry*, 149, 654–658.

Wode-Helgodt, B., Berg, G., Petterson, U., Rydelius, P.A. and Trollehed, H. (1988) Group therapy with schizophrenic patients in outpatient departments. *Acta Psychiatrica Scandinavica*, 78, 304–313.

Wykes, T., Steel, C., Everitt, B., and Tarrier, N. (2008) Cognitive behavior therapy for schizophrenia: Effect sizes, clinical models, and methodological rigor. *Schizophrenia Bulletin*, 34, 523–537.

Xia, J., Merinder, L.B. and Belgamwar, M.R. (2011) Psychoeducation for schizophrenia. *Schizophrenia Bulletin*, 37, 21–22.

4 Clinical Issues of the Integrative Model
The Basics

Introduction

In this and the next chapter, clinical issues related to conducting groups for psychotic patients using the *integrative* model will be discussed. Major points will be illustrated by brief clinical vignettes, and in this chapter, a description of a typical session will be given. Hopefully, the reader will pick up enough clinical points to conduct his or her own group in a variety of settings, from inpatient, to time-limited outpatient, to long-term outpatient.

Background

In my book on group therapy with schizophrenic patients, I used the term "integrative" to describe my empirically derived treatment model that borrowed from psychoeducational, psychodynamic, and interpersonal approaches (Kanas, 1996). Over the years, some cognitive-behavioral therapy (CBT) components have become incorporated into the model.

The impetus for the integrative approach stemmed from a large study I conducted while serving in the United States Air Force during the post-Viet Nam period (Kanas et al., 1978, 1980). The setting was a general psychiatric unit at a large United States Air Force teaching hospital. The patients were active duty personnel, dependents, and military retirees. All newly admitted patients to the unit who signed informed consent were randomly assigned to participate in one of three conditions, given three times per week for one hour: general group therapy, activities-oriented group therapy, or free time on the ward. The therapy group followed an insight-oriented, uncovering approach taken from psychoanalytic theory that encouraged the expression of affects. This approach was commonly used at that time for non-psychotic patients, and since our group included both psychotic and non-psychotic members, it formed the basis for the treatment. Patients were evaluated at admission and after eight experimental days (about 20 total days of hospitalization) by nurse evaluators who were blind to experimental condition. Outcome measures included the Psychiatric Evaluation Form and the Global Assessment Scale. Patient medication usage and individual therapy contact minutes were recorded.

A total of 86 patients participated (63% male and 44% psychotic—nearly all schizophrenic). The majority of patients improved overall, and there were no significant differences in improvement rates among the three conditions (Kanas et al., 1980). However, significantly more psychotic patients in the group therapy condition scored *worse* on our clinical measures than psychotic patients in the other two conditions. There were no worsening effects of the group for the nonpsychotic patients. So, it seemed that the group approach that encouraged insight, uncovering, and affect expression was toxic for acutely psychotic patients compared with a supportive activities group and no group.

After leaving the Air Force and taking a position at the San Francisco Department of Veterans Affairs Medical Center (SFVA) in 1977, I started experimenting with a clinical model that might better meet the needs of psychotic patients. I decided that a safe, supportive approach that focused on psychotic symptoms and relationship issues was best. I conceived of a model that took appropriate aspects from psychodynamic, psychoeducational, and interpersonal theory and techniques that was specially designed with the needs of psychotic patients in mind. I called it an *integrative* approach. Similarly, techniques that seemed harmful (such as anxiety-producing silences, activation of unconscious conflicts, and the encouragement of strong affects) were not to be encouraged. The treatment model was begun on a general psychiatric unit at the SFVA, and it led to a series of outcome and process studies, both in the inpatient and later in the outpatient setting. These studies will be reviewed in Chapter 6. In this chapter and the next, the clinical model will be presented, along with clinical vignettes to assist the reader.

But first, it should be noted that in recent years, the term "integrative" has been used to describe evidence-based approaches residing more in the didactic camp (i.e., involving psychoeducational and cognitive-behavioral approaches, including social skills training and multi-family therapy). However, Pearson and Burlingame (2013) have pointed out that recent research on group treatments for difficult to treat patients (including those with schizophrenia) has led to "integrative group treatment protocols that combine CBT and other structured group protocols with more traditional psychodynamic...or process groups" (p. 607). I agree with this sentiment.

In what follows, I will define my *integrative* group treatment model as *an evidence-based, group therapeutic approach that uses clinical principles that combine both non-didactic (psychodynamic and interpersonal) and didactic (psychoeducational and cognitive-behavioral) techniques into one coordinated treatment model.*

Clinical Limitations of Non-integrative Approaches

Taken alone, each of the four main approaches that contribute to the model have continued to be used; but in their pure forms, they have some disadvantages. The psychoeducational and CBT models often do not pay enough attention to the interpersonal needs of these isolated patients, and their lecture format may not allow enough time for corrections to be made in maladaptive interactions observed in the here-and-now of the sessions. Also, the presence of a planned lecture sequence does not allow enough flexibility to deal with crises and topic areas that may be of special interest to the patients attending the group that day. The psychoanalytic/psychodynamic approach can deal with such issues, but too much emphasis on insight, transference, and regression may uncover unpleasant unconscious memories and affects that produce anxiety. Too much anxiety and regression has been found to exacerbate psychotic symptoms in schizophrenic patients (Drake and Sederer, 1986; Geczy and Sultenfuss, 1995; Kanas et al., 1980; MacDonald, Blochberger and Maynard, 1964; Pattison, Brissenden and Wohl, 1967; Strassberg et al., 1975; Weiner, 1984). In addition, transference-oriented interpretations have not been terribly useful with severely mentally ill patients (Kapur, 1993), and the psychoanalytic/psychodynamic model does not emphasize the here-and-now as much as events that occurred in the past. The interpersonal approach does, but at the risk of short-changing issues related to coping with symptoms, strengthening ego functions, and discussing psychological problems concerning non-relationship issues. Also, like too much uncovering, the here-and-now focus can at times be too intensive, particularly around affect expression, and it can lead to anxiety and regression during the group sessions.

The Integrative Model: An Overview

Before discussing specific issues related to my integrative model, I want to say a few words about the value of coping with symptoms, an important component. Like other people with chronic medical conditions, most people with chronic psychotic disorders will not be "cured" of their illness (i.e., become totally symptom-free). Rather, with the use of medication and the therapeutic techniques discussed below, they will learn to control their symptoms, so that they are minimized or at least tolerated to the point of improving the patient's functionality and ability to relate better with others. Most people need help to do this before they can develop successful coping strategies.

Robert Francis has described how he has dealt with the symptoms of his chronic schizophrenia:

> Twenty plus years into the illness, now while I'm experiencing multiple symptoms, I have a definite strategy. I now closely monitor, observe, and regulate my behavior and my conversations, and I make sure that I am acting as rationally, routine, and of the mindset of "minding my own business" while doing my best to engage in

"everyday" behaviors, including engaging in benign and superficial conversations. I monitor my behavior, actions, and words for reasons of personal sustenance. Doing this allows me to continue to function as an ordinary citizen. It allows me to work, drive, do my errands, socialize, and in general participate in the consensus reality of society.

(Francis, 2019, p. 45)

As a licensed clinical social worker, Francis has been a success story in his ability to function despite ongoing psychotic symptoms. But it has not been easy for him, and he has to work hard every day to cope with his psychosis and still be a productive member of society.

Psychodynamic Issues

As mentioned above, my integrative group therapy treatment model borrows from four schools of thought: psychodynamic, interpersonal, CBT, and psychoeducational. Issues related to the psychodynamic approach are shown in Table 4.1. Here, the focus is on psychological problems facing the patients. This focus is approached through patient-generated discussions, where the group members set the agenda for the sessions so long as the topics are consistent with the group goals. This allows a patient with an urgent issue to express him- or herself without fear of interrupting a pre-set agenda, and it contributes to the sense that the group belongs to the patients rather than to the therapists. Although presentations from the therapist occasionally may be given as part of the psychoeducational or CBT component (see below), they are rare. The only formal agenda items that occur are related to introducing a new member into the group or saying goodbye to an old member or therapist who is leaving (see below). At the beginning of most sessions, patients are asked what they want to talk about today, or how their week went. If a long

Table 4.1 Integrative model: psychodynamic issues

Issue	Examples
Emphasis:	Psychological problems
Goals:	Understand psychotic triggers
	Gain insight into relevant long-term maladaptive developmental patterns
Aims:	Focus on improving reality sense
	Examine factors that make symptoms better or worse
	Examine the roll of long-standing problems and maladaptive patterns of relating on current functioning (typically after 4–6 months)
Techniques:	Patient-generated discussions
	Sharing life stories with other group members
	Interpreting metaphors

silence ensues, the group leader might ask each patient to review his week via a formal go-around (where each member takes a turn in speaking). Occasionally, the leader may prime the pump by suggesting a topic, but this is uncommon.

Psychological goals relate to enumerating factors that make the symptoms of the psychosis better or worse. Later in the life of the group, when trust has been established and patients are comfortable with each other (typically, around four to six months), the effects of long-term maladaptive patterns of behavior on current symptoms may be considered, such as the effects of years of mistrust based on abusive parenting or suspicion of others based on childhood bullying. Fine-tuning the ability to sense reality may be discussed as well as the appropriateness of one's belief system. For example, feeling suspicious of strangers while walking in a dangerous neighborhood at night is reason for concern in most people, whereas feeling the same way at a church function during the daytime is likely not a good interpretation of reality. Since the belief systems of psychotic people often are locked up in biased and rigid thinking patterns, they tend to interpret the reality of events the same regardless of the situation, and they need to learn to be more three-dimensional in their approach to the world.

Stone (1996) has pointed out the value of interpreting metaphors in groups of chronically mentally ill patients. He states:

> Much communication takes place via metaphors. Patients respond to a stimulus that evokes affect (either consciously or unconsciously), and they comment upon their feelings through metaphors. The most difficult feelings for patients to manage are those stimulated in the transferences and here-and-now interactions within the group. The therapist's tasks are to 'hear' and understand the communication and decide in what manner to intervene.
>
> (Stone, p. 108)

The following vignette illustrates this point from one of my groups:

> Vignette 4.1. A schizophrenic outpatient named A came into the group and began talking about an altercation he experienced on the bus whereby a woman started harassing the driver and then another person nearby. He wanted to intervene, but he held his temper for fear that he would be harmed or lose control. Thinking that this event was a metaphor for his psychotic condition, one of the coleaders of the group pointed out that recently in the news, there were reports of mass shootings in Gilroy, California, El Paso, Texas, and Dayton, Ohio. He asked the patient if he was feeling vulnerable about his illness and feeling threatened "out there." The patient responded by saying yes, he was worried about his safety and losing control,

possibly harming someone or decompensating into further psychosis. This led to a general discussion of impulse control and vulnerability felt by other group patients due to their psychotic condition.

Stone also mentions that metaphors may result in a displacement of strong feelings that may result from the group, such as a therapist's absence or the introduction of a new member, and that the group leaders must be aware of this issue. In Vignette 4.1, however, the most likely triggers were external to the group process.

In Chapter 2, I discussed the notion of ego functions as part of the psychodynamic tradition. Two notions that are especially relevant for groups of psychotic patients are reality sense and reality testing. Being made conscious of the fact that what one perceives as real may not be so is important for people with schizophrenia spectrum disorders. In this way, a sense that what one perceives is not real can be followed by actions to test out these perceptions. Since reality testing is closely tied to coping with psychotic symptoms, it will be discussed later.

Uncovering techniques, such as the use of free associations, actively exploring the unconscious, or interpreting transference, are used rarely in the integrative group, since they may produce anxiety and regression in psychotic patients. Similarly, the expression of strong affects during the sessions is not encouraged for the same reasons. At times, these strong emotions need to be diverted into more manageable channels:

> Vignette 4.2. Patient B in an inpatient group became annoyed at patient C. He raised his voice and began to berate him, which caused C to recoil and raised the anxiety level in the room (as manifested by jittery movements and worried looks in the other group members). The leader intervened, saying that it sounded like B was reacting to something C had said rather than to him personally, and he reframed the interaction in these terms. B agreed, and the discussion switched into how what people say can offend others and how we can learn to be more diplomatic in our comments. By labelling the affect in less personal terms, the therapist was able to defuse the anxiety and focus on a behavior rather than an issue of personalities.

Unlike groups of non-psychotic patients, where the expression of strong affects may be encouraged, it is important for groups of psychotic patients to be safe and for affects to be modulated to prevent strong feelings from erupting. Psychotic egos are fragile and poorly defended, and too much affect may result in overwhelming anxiety. The damage done to psychotic patients in the Air Force study presented at the beginning of this chapter likely was due to poor attention to this issue.

Interpersonal Issues

Important interpersonal issues used in the integrative group therapy model are shown in Table 4.2. Here, the major goal is to improve interpersonal relationships, both in the area of forming new relationships and then maintaining them over time. This is done in the group in two ways. First, many group topics relate to meeting new people, breaking the ice, tolerating social events, and putting oneself in a situation for interpersonal success. For example, if a patient is religious or has a hobby (such as chess or stamps), he or she is encouraged to go to church or join a club focusing on this hobby. In this way, safe relationships may form based on the common interest. Patients also are encouraged to interact with each other outside the group around such interests:

> Vignette 4.3. Patient D in an outpatient group for schizophrenic patients stated in passing that he had a pool table in his house and loved to play. Patient E and others also expressed an interest in pool. The therapist commented that perhaps they could all get together for a pool game. Patient D invited them all to come to his house. The therapist encouraged this and suggested they do so and report back to the group. The next session, only E had taken D up on his offer. It went well for these two, who reported having had a nice time.

Note that extra-group contact was encouraged, with the proviso that the event be reported back to the group. Group members, especially at a Veterans Affair hospital, sometimes will socialize over coffee before the group session or give each other rides to the clinic. It is important that all extra-group contacts between patients, however encouraged, be brought back into the group for discussion and comment by the therapist and other patients.

Table 4.2 Integrative model: interpersonal issues

Issue	*Examples*
Emphasis:	Interpersonal problems
Goals:	Form and maintain improved relationships with other people
Aims:	Discuss relationship problems
	Practice healthy interactions in the here-and-now of the group
Techniques:	Patient-generated discussions
	Pointing out positive and negative interactions in the here-and-now of the group
	In-group practice of eye contact and relating with other group members
	Role-playing
	Extra-group contact, provided the event is discussed in the next group session

A second way that interpersonal issues are considered is in the here-and-now of the group process. Making observations of how people interact during the sessions is an important aspect of groups based on the interpersonal approach, and it can be a powerful change factor. Patients can learn from both positive and negative interactions. Role-playing a different way of interacting sometimes can be useful as well. Even small bits of relation-oriented behaviors are addressed, such as making eye contact:

> Vignette 4.4. Patient F in an outpatient group started talking about how patient G could improve his relationships, while at the same time looking at the therapist while making his comments. The therapist interrupted him by saying: "I think you are talking about G. Why don't you look at him?" F began doing so, but then started looking at the therapist again. The therapist took his finger and pointed at G. F immediately got the hint and looked back at G. When F finished talking, the therapist congratulated him for his "great input" and asked G how it felt to be addressed and looked at directly. He said he liked it. This led to a discussion about the importance of eye contact in initiating and maintaining interactions with other people.

Psychotic patients often have problems with eye contact. Sometimes, they fantasize that someone looking at them directly may be intending to do them harm or may "penetrate into my soul" through their eyes. For this reason, some patients look away or wear sun glasses to avoid eye contact. These fears sometimes form the basis of a group discussion topic, such as the difference between staring and oogling versus casually making eye contact in an effort to engage someone else. We also might discuss environments where avoiding eye contact is a socially condoned behavior, such as on buses or in gyms.

The here-and-now of the group also can be used to help patients deal with symptoms, especially when they exhibit the symptom during the session (see Vignette 4.6, below). This doesn't always result in an "a-ha" revelation, but it usually sets the stage for future discussions of psychotic experiences and the way that we can learn to test their reality, such as asking other people if they experience the same thing.

Although group members are encouraged to interact and give each other advice about problems, if this seems to raise the anxiety level during the session, the therapist may take over and give his or her own advice to take the pressure away from the group members. As with all here-and-now interventions, therapists must titrate the anxiety level of the intervention, which typically is more powerful than discussions of issues related to the past or to people outside of the group (i.e., there-and-then situations).

CBT Issues

Important CBT issues used in the integrative model are shown in Table 4.3. The main goals here relate to reframing cognitive distortions and practicing coping behaviors to deal with symptoms. The main targets are hallucinations, delusions, and loose associations. In order to cope with such symptoms, some reality testing ability is necessary. It is useful to discuss this issue with a presentation of the A–B–C model:

> Vignette 4.5. In an outpatient group, H was having problems understanding why he misinterpreted things in his life. The therapist got out his marking pen and wrote on a white board: "A (antecedents or causes)—B (beliefs or biases)—C (consequences or behaviors)." Under "B," he listed a number of distortions people have of the world, such as: nothing changes, so it is OK to jump to the same conclusion; blaming problems on others; and perceiving the world as a dangerous place. He then discussed how internal problems may be attributed to the outside (e.g., vulnerable feelings become the delusion that people are out to get you; threatening inner voices become scary auditory hallucinations; poor self-esteem is turned into compensatory grandiosity). He further explained that these distortions become fixed into beliefs that may be used no matter what the situation. Finally, he discussed how our beliefs affect our behaviors (i.e., have consequences), and how our behaviors feedback to influence how we believe about similar events in the future. This presentation helped H visually understand the role that his distorted ideas played in complicating his life, and it led the group into a general discussion about faulty beliefs.

Table 4.3 Integrative model: cognitive-behavioral issues

Issue	Examples
Emphasis:	Cognitive distortions and psychotic symptoms
Goals:	Reframe thinking
	Share successful coping strategies
Aims:	Discuss ways of reality testing
	Learn strategies of coping with hallucinations, delusions, and loose associations
Techniques:	White board presentations (A–B–C model, vulnerability-stress model)
	Advice-giving from leaders and patients
	Role-playing
	In-group practice
	Homework

As mentioned in Chapter 2, the A–B–C model also helps patients test reality by employing strategies for coping with psychotic experiences:

> Vignette 4.6. Patient I in an inpatient group began mumbling to himself and looking around. The therapist asked him if he was hearing voices. The patient said yes. The therapist then asked him to describe the voices, which it turned out were persecutory in nature and related to his feeling threatened by people on the ward. The therapist then asked other group members if they heard the same voices. All of them said no, although a couple acknowledged that sometimes they heard their own voices coming from outside their heads. The therapist then asked patient I if perhaps the voices he heard were generated by his own mind. He was not entirely convinced, but he admitted that maybe this was the case. The therapist then suggested that if the voices were generated by his mind, perhaps what they said about the ward was not true. Other group members said they felt safe on the ward. The therapist linked these revelations to the patient learning ways of coping better with these voices in the future. Various coping strategies were suggested by other group members (e.g., asking friends or family members if they too heard or believed the content of the voices he was hearing; noting if what the voices said actually reflected future events; doing an activity to focus his mind away from the voices; taking a prescribed extra dose of medication). Patient I later reported that he employed some of these techniques outside of the group and felt more comfortable on the ward, despite continuing to hear voices.

The vulnerability-stress model also is useful in showing patients the relationship between our makeup and how we deal with external stressors:

> Vignette 4.7. In an outpatient group, patient J described a variety of ways that problems in his life (e.g., low income, bad housing, stigma of mental illness) exacerbated his symptoms. The group leader wrote on a white board two columns, one labeled "vulnerability" and the other "stressors." Under the first, he listed genetic makeup, neurodevelopmental and neurocognitive status, and biased thinking. Under the second, he listed life events, daily hassles, and social stressors. He explained that our inherent psychological vulnerabilities interact with stressors in life to cause stress which, left untreated, can precipitate the symptoms of psychosis in some people, but in others, anxiety or depression or high blood pressure. If treated with medications, individual or group therapy, family support, and social skills training, the interaction of vulnerability and stressors may result in no or milder symptoms. J liked this description and began to examine factors he could affect through treatment to compensate for his vulnerabilities.

White board exercises such as these are useful, not only in helping patients understand their illness better, but also stimulating a common language for future discussions about coping strategies. I try to include an A–B–C and vulnerability-stress presentation in the life of every group, usually when an issue comes up that is related to these two notions. Some therapists may want to present them formally early in the life of a group, but I think they are more powerful and better accepted if presented in the context of a relevant discussion.

Patients learn coping strategies from each other, with encouragement from the group leaders. Some patients experience a quieting of their voices if they go into a secluded area and yell or swear at them to go away. Another coping strategy is to use ear phones and play quiet music or have no sound at all (as if the ear phones block the voices from the outside). Another set of coping strategies relates to a high/low stress model, which will be discussed in the next section.

Cognitive reframing also can be useful:

> Vignette 4.8. In an outpatient group, K described feeling angry and depressed about paying a large cleaning deposit to an old landlord when he moved into a much better apartment. The group leader asked K to describe some of the advantages of the new apartment, of which there were many (e.g., lower rent, friendlier neighbors, better location). The therapist then said that dwelling on the cleaning deposit was looking at a glass half empty, when in fact moving into a better place was like looking at a glass half full. K understood the metaphor and brightened up, saying he felt better about the total situation.

Most schizophrenia spectrum people think concretely and have trouble with metaphors and other abstract thinking, but K was able to grasp the meaning of the therapist, and he and the other group members could observe how approaching a problem in a different way could improve one's mood.

Psychoeducational Issues

Psychoeducation also plays a role in the integrative model, as shown in Table 4.4. The main goals are to help the patients better understand the biological nature of their disease and some of its treatment considerations. Brief verbal or white board presentations of causes, symptoms, course, and treatment can be given. Usually, these presentations are prompted by the group discussion rather than being organized as a series of lectures. In this way, they have more relevance for the patients and do not sabotage the value of letting the patients set the agenda and focus on their interpersonal interactions in the here-and-now.

Table 4.4 Integrative model: psychoeducational issues

Issue	Examples
Emphasis:	Biological and phenomenological aspects of psychotic diseases
Goals:	Understand the nature of the disease and its treatment
Aims:	Learn about disease causes, symptoms, course, and treatment
Techniques:	White board presentations ("U" curve external stimulation-symptom relationship)
	Relaxation exercises
	Advice-giving from leader
	Question and answer discussions
	Homework

One of my favorite psychoeducational topics is to visually show the relationship between external stimulation and symptoms:

> Vignette 4.9. In an outpatient group, L talked about feeling anxious when he was asked to give a talk at his rehabilitation program graduation. He also said that he felt anxious in other high-profile situations, and that during these times his voices would get louder. The therapist presented the notion that external stimulation can lead to an exacerbation of hallucinations, but L seemed to miss the point. The therapist then went to a white board and drew a graph with a large "U" on it. He labeled the horizontal axis "stimulation," with "low" marked to the left and "high" marked to the right. The vertical axis was labelled "symptom (voices)," with "low" at the bottom and "high" at the top. The graph showed that under conditions of low or high external stimulation, the ends of the "U" resulted in more prominent hallucinations (i.e., high values on the "voices" axis), whereas under moderate conditions of stimulation, the middle of the "U," hallucinations were relatively quiet. This visual presentation led to a general discussion of how people like to operate under moderate external stimulation, whereas very low or very high stimulation can result in anxiety and exacerbation of psychotic symptoms.

One offshoot of this approach is to treat symptoms of mental disease as analogous to symptoms of a medical disease, such as high blood pressure. For example, the therapist can point out that stress can cause increased blood pressure in people prone to hypertension, anxiety or depression in non-psychotic people, and louder voices in those with a predisposition to psychosis. Analogies like these tend to reduce stigma and place psychotic symptoms in a continuum with other medical conditions.

Occasionally, relaxation techniques may be practiced in the group, and the theoretical reasoning behind these can be presented briefly:

> Vignette 4.10. In an outpatient group, M talked about feeling anxious, and another patient responded by telling him about an approach he learned to systematically relax the major muscle groups in his body by first tensing them, then relaxing them one by one, starting with his legs and working up. The group members practiced doing this during the session. The therapist then mentioned the value for some in diaphragmatic breathing. He said that the gut contains a great deal of serotonin, a neurotransmitter that can help people relax. By breathing with the diaphragm rather than with the chest muscles, there was some evidence that a person could stimulate serotonin release. He had the group members link their hands behind the back of the chair, close their eyes, and focus on breathing from their abdomen for a minute. He then asked if they felt more relaxed, and many said yes. He summarized that both of these simple non-medical exercises could be used in a variety of settings outside the group to quell anxiety.

Other relaxation activities, such as meditation, also can be tried in the group, although it might be a better use of group time to refer patients to a gym or school, where they can learn better meditative practices.

The same goes for other therapeutic activities, such as medications and social services. Although the importance of these treatment methods can be discussed and shared in the group, especially the value of taking medications, the therapist must be mindful to not use too much group time discussing these subjects in great detail (e.g., medication dosages, specific halfway houses). Patients can get this information elsewhere, such as in a medication clinic or a social work referral, or in a homework reading assignment. The main issues of the integrative group rarely are discussed elsewhere, and precious group time needs to focus on such topics.

Group Goals

There are two major goals for integrative groups. One is to help patients identify and learn strategies of coping with psychotic experiences, such as hallucinations, delusions, and disorganized thinking. Negative symptoms also are addressed. The second major goal is to help the patients form and maintain healthier interpersonal relationships with others. This is done not only through the *content* of the group discussions, but also in the group *process*, where patients are encouraged to practice interacting with others during the sessions in real time (i.e., in the here-and-now) by directing comments to them and maintaining good eye contact. The idea is to create a safe environment, where the patients can openly discuss their psychotic and interpersonal problems and share ways of dealing with them with people who have experienced similar issues. A mantra that is recited from time to time in the group, especially when there are new patients or cotherapists, is the following: *this is a group for people who have had nervous breakdowns—we discuss issues such as hearing voices, feeling suspicious, being confused, or having problems relating with other people.*

As we shall see below, the emphasis on one goal or another may depend upon the setting and stages of the group. Also, in long-term groups, typically after four to six months, long-standing problems and maladaptive patterns of relating with others may be discussed as well. But even in these sessions, the leaders must be mindful that such discussions should be related to the two main group goals affecting the patients in the present: coping with psychotic symptoms and improving interpersonal relationships.

Typical Sequence of Events in a Session

A typical session proceeds as follows in terms of the topic to be discussed:

Identification → *Generalization* → *Coping*

In most sessions, the therapist begins with either no comment or something vague, such as "How is everyone today?" or "What do you want to talk about?" Patients are encouraged to come up with a topic area that is relevant to the group goals (unless, of course, something ominous is raised that takes precedence, such as suicidal or homicidal ideation—see Chapter 5). When an appropriate topic is raised, such as "My voices have been worse this week" or "I had a fight with my friend," the group leader expresses interest, since now someone in the group has *identified* a relevant topic. The therapist may then explore it a bit to tease out some of the details.

Then the leader explores whether or not this topic is of interest to the other group members. By *generalizing* it, the therapist takes stock as to whether or not the members present in the group that day can relate to the topic and can share ideas about it. The group leader may ask the members if anyone else has experienced this as a problem, and if no one comments, the leader can conduct a formal go-around, where all patients are asked to comment in turn. After all the patients have been given a chance to speak, the group leader evaluates whether or not enough of the group members can relate to the topic at hand, or if another topic should be proposed. In the latter case, the leader might suggest a related topic, or he or she might ask the members if another topic might be discussed that has broader interest that day.

Once a topic has been decided upon, the group enters the phase where the members are asked to share *coping* strategies. This phase should occupy at least half of the session time. Patient input is more important than therapist input. This can be encouraged in two ways: directing the issue to the group-as-a-whole or using a member with the problem as the focal point. For example, if auditory hallucination is the topic, the leader might say something like "It sounds like many of you have had problems dealing with voices. What strategies have you found useful to deal with them?" (or "to make them quieter?"). Then the therapist can look down or away from the group members, hoping that the ensuing silence will stimulate someone to speak. Alternatively, the therapist can use the person first bringing up the topic as a focus for discussion, such as "John is having problems coping with his voices. Can anyone give him some advice?" If no one comments, the therapist might ask a specific patient to help John: "Sarah, you say you have had some difficulties with your voices. Can you tell John what works for you?" The key is to encourage the patients to interact around advice related to coping strategies, with good eye contact. This serves not only the coping agenda, but also the agenda of practicing good interpersonal interactions in the here-and-now of the group.

Clinical Illustration of a Typical Session

To illustrate some of these points, I will describe a typical session. This was session number 6 from a 12-session, time-limited outpatient therapy group. Present were six patients (five male, one female), all schizophrenia spectrum, and a cotherapy team consisting of a female psychology student and a male staff psychiatrist (Dr. K). The names of all participants have been altered.

> Bill began the session by announcing: "I'm in a crisis...I have emphysema," which was a recent diagnosis. He admitted that it was a mild case, then after a pause proceeded to ask Jim how much he spends at a local fast food restaurant. This led to a general discussion about food costs. In an effort to direct the group to a topic consistent with the group goals of coping with psychotic symptoms and relating better with other people, Dr. K asked Bill how he felt about his crisis. Bill said he wasn't too worried, then started talking about the cost of housing. Cotherapist Ms. Davis asked the group if anyone was worried about their health. Evan said he had high blood pressure, and others alluded to similar medical problems. Seeing that the group was stuck, Dr. K pointedly asked them: "How about your mental disease?" Bill then said: "I have weird thoughts...my mind wanders." Evan, Ron and Jim looked at Bill and described similar experiences. Dr. K then did a go-around to ask the remaining members if they too had a similar problem with their thoughts wandering. Jake said he did, but Elaine said her mind did not wander. Seeing that all the patients acknowledged loose associations except for Elaine, and wanting her to be included in the discussion, he asked her if she could give

the "fellas" advice about how to cope with their wandering thoughts. She said "discipline" worked for her: she was able to discipline her thinking so that her mind didn't wander so much. Dr. K then asked the other members how they coped with their mind wandering and other mental problems, and several ideas were expressed, such as taking more antipsychotic medication; watching television or reading a book to take their minds off of intrusive thoughts; and talking to themselves when they heard voices, telling them to go away. Dr. K pointed out to Bill how his mind had wandered during the session, such as when he started talking about his physical crisis, then suddenly jumped to food prices, then to housing costs. Dr. K asked if it would be helpful for him to learn to stop talking after completing one idea so that he would not drift off to another. Bill said yes. Dr. K. asked him if he minded being interrupted by one of the group leaders in future sessions after completing a thought so that he could practice focusing better, and he said he wouldn't mind. (This was done in subsequent sessions.)

Dr. K then asked the group members to consider what made their mental symptoms worse, and several patients commented that stress from family members exacerbated their symptoms. Elaine talked about problems she had relating to her daughter, Bill acknowledged having problems with his sister, and Ron described general family stressors. In contrast, Evan said that he received support from his wife, who helped him deal with day to day stress. This led to a discussion about the difficulties some of the patients had in trusting other people. Bill said the only person he trusts is legally blind and that he was still holding a grudge with someone about something that happened 17 years ago. He also alluded to general family problems. Ms. Davis offered her opinion that it helps to talk things over and get support from people you trust.

After a pause, Evan asked the members about their income, and Elaine mentioned the high cost of an apartment. Dr. K pointed out that the group was drifting off topic again. He commented that Bill had many stressors from dealing with other people and asked if anyone else had this experience. Jake said he did, and he described problems he has with his mother controlling what he eats. He said he expressed his independence the previous week by having a milkshake on his own, and he credited this to a suggestion made by Ron during the previous session that he should do more for himself. Dr. K asked Ron how he felt about helping Jake, and Ron smiled. Dr. K said that it was important for people to treat themselves occasionally with favorite foods or fun activities, such as hobbies, especially those that involved other people. Jake said that he has no friends where he lives and feels controlled by his mother and step-father. Elaine suggested he make friends. Dr. K reinforced this idea and suggested that the group members could socialize between sessions for a movie or a meal and report on this experience in the group. Time was up, and the session ended.

Several points can be made about this session. It is ideal for patients to discuss experiences related to psychotic symptoms or relationship problems and give each other feedback about ways to cope with them. In this group, the members began by disjointedly discussing a number of topics, such as restaurants, housing, and medical issues, that were not related to the group goals. Subtle comments made by the group leaders that were aimed to focus the members on more appropriate topics were ignored, and it was only when Dr. K asked them point blank about their mental disease that they began to focus on this area. Although usually just one relevant topic is mentioned at the beginning of a session, here there were two: weird thoughts (i.e., delusions) and mind wandering (i.e., loose associations). Dr. K decided to focus on only one: loose associations.

During the generalization phase of the session, Elaine was the only one not admitting to having this problem. In order for her not to be singled out and possibly scapegoated as the only person not having loose associations (and being the only woman patient), Dr. K involved her in the discussion by asking her to give feedback to the others. The members gave each other helpful coping advice and maintained good eye contact in the process. Dr. K also asked permission to tell a patient when he was drifting off topic, which is a good here-and-now behavioral method of training people to deal with loose associations.

After a general discussion of coping strategies for thinking and associative problems, there was enough time left to bring up another topic: how family and other interpersonal stressors can exacerbate symptoms. Since several group members said familial issues were a problem for them, strategies for coping with such stressors were discussed, along with the suggestion that the patients make new friends. As members of a therapy group learn to trust one another, they can be encouraged to interact socially between sessions, provided that they bring their experiences back to the group. Sometimes, they can be given specific homework for the week after a session. Although Dr. K gave the members permission to socialize outside of the group, explicit homework to do this was not prescribed in this session (but see Vignette 4.3).

Patient Inclusion/Exclusion

I have found diagnosis to be a useful construct in setting up groups with psychotic patients, using the standard criteria described in Chapter 1. For most integrative groups, the patients are in the schizophrenia spectrum (e.g., schizophrenia, schizoaffective disorder, delusional disorder), or they chronically experience prominent psychotic symptoms or signs most of the time that they want help with. For example, a few non-acute bipolar patients continue to have lingering grandiosity or rapid thoughts, and if they want to address these, they may be admitted to the group. Also, patients with questionable diagnoses (e.g., Psychosis Not Otherwise Specified) who experience hallucinations or delusions may be included, provided they experience such symptoms chronically. The same goes for severely depressed patients whose despair and self-esteem reach psychotic proportions. A special integrative model for treating euthymic bipolar patients without psychotic symptoms is the subject of Chapter 7.

Many people with acute psychosis related to stress, substance abuse, medication side effects, medical illness, or borderline personality decompensation usually don't become involved with integrative psychosis groups. This is because their psychosis is transient, and during most of their lives, such symptoms are not an issue. People with non-psychotic depressions or personality disorders don't relate to most of the issues discussed in integrative groups (other than relationship issues), and they should be referred to other therapy groups that better meet their needs, such as those focusing on insight, affect expression, and the uncovering of traumatic unconscious issues. Other patients who are not admitted include those who don't benefit from any talking form of group therapy (e.g., those with severe dementia, such as Alzheimer's disease), those who consciously try to disrupt or sabotage the group for the other group members (e.g., patients with severe antisocial disorder), and those who are overstimulated by any group activity (e.g., acute manic patients).

Homogeneous versus Heterogeneous Groups

The cohesiveness of any therapy group is positively affected by how homogeneous it is in terms of the patients who are participating. What is meant by "homogeneous" is relative, however, since it is a concept that can be expressed in terms of many different parameters, such as diagnosis, cognitive functioning, ability to relate interpersonally, symptomatology, etc. As indicated in the previous section, most psychosis integrative groups are composed of patients with schizophrenia spectrum disorder or difficulties where psychotic symptoms are continuing and problematic.

Putting patients with psychosis in homogeneous groups has several advantages. First, since they have much in common, they can relate quickly to each other's problems. This rapid development of cohesiveness especially is useful in settings where the patients can only attend a limited number of sessions, such as in the inpatient setting or in brief, time-limited outpatient groups. Second, specific clinical techniques can be employed which are designed for the needs of this particular type of patient. For example, an approach that focuses on coping strategies for psychotic symptoms would be quite relevant for a group discussion involving schizophrenic patients, whereas it might be inappropriate and boring for group members who had never before experienced a break in reality (such as people with personality disorders). Finally, techniques can be avoided that might be harmful for psychotic patients. For example, clinical strategies that try to stimulate the emergence of unconscious material (e.g., long silences, emphasis on past conflicts) or encourage the expression of anger and other strong emotions in the group may be useful for patients with depression or personality disorders, but they may produce anxiety and regression in psychotic patients that may increase their symptoms.

Despite these clinical advantages, there may be a practical problem in establishing a homogeneous psychotic group in some inpatient and outpatient settings. For example, there may not be enough patients on the ward or in the clinic at a given time to form a group for psychotic patients. In such cases, one must consider forming a group with patients from two (or possibly more) wards or clinics, which is workable, provided that the staff from these different settings communicate with one another and ensure that all the patients attend. It also helps if they communicate special problems to the group leader or, in groups using a cotherapy approach, if each of the leaders is from one of the participating programs.

Where homogeneous integrative groups are not possible, heterogeneous mixtures of psychotic and non-psychotic patients may be tried, although for the reasons mentioned in the previous section, such groups are not ideal. In inpatient settings, these groups may consist of the patients and therapists from the same treatment team (Yalom, 1983). In outpatient settings, the heterogeneous approach works best when all the patients are clinically stable and can tolerate some degree of anxiety and regression. This usually results in a format that is supportive and focuses on current problems. These groups generally are found in clinics dealing with the chronically mentally ill. The non-psychotic patients in such integrative groups generally are low-functioning and suffer from severe depression, personality disorders, or other chronic mental conditions. These individuals can be helpful to psychotic patients by providing them with reality-based advice and relatively undistorted feedback concerning hallucinations, delusions, and meeting new people. All group members can relate to general symptoms like despair over having a chronic mental condition, to societal stigma prompted by their serious mental disease, or to maladaptive interpersonal relationships, so there is some common ground.

Group Format Issues

Format issues for integrative groups are shown in Table 4.5. These are recommended parameters; therapists should take their own staffing and setting into account when forming such groups. It is useful to discuss inpatient and outpatient group separately.

Table 4.5 Group format issues: integrative groups

Issue	Inpatient groups	Outpatient groups
Sessions per week	3–5	1–2
Duration of session	45 minutes	45–90 minutes
Type of group	Open	Closed or slow-open
Number of therapists	2	1–2
Enrolled patients	6–8	6–10
Ideal number of patients in a session	5–6	6–8

Inpatient Groups

Inpatient groups typically have new patients entering or discharged patients leaving during each session, and such groups are called *open* groups. Time must be set aside to introduce a new patient or say goodbye to a departing member in this setting. Because of this ongoing turnover, it is hard for inpatient groups to form cohesive units, where patients get to know and trust each other. Also, clinical status varies greatly in the group, with a new patient often exhibiting acute psychosis with active and disturbing hallucinations or delusions, and sometimes needing to leave a session as a result. Given such disruptions, it is useful to cap the number of patients at eight and the duration for each session at 45 minutes. In addition, it is recommended to have two group leaders, since sometimes one will need to leave the group with a disturbed or disruptive patient to calm them down or get some medication. This will allow the other to remain in the group to continue the session or process the disturbance with the remaining members. Should the patient return, he or she should be welcomed back into the group and asked how he or she is now feeling before continuing the session.

If there are only two patients in the group, the therapists have the option of splitting them up and conducting supportive individual sessions or continuing using the group format.

If there are three or more patients, then the therapists should proceed using the group format. Groups of four or fewer patients require the leaders to be more active, since the opportunities for patient-to-patient interactions are low, and the therapists may have to become "pseudo-group members" and offer their opinions as they lead the discussion. These very small group sessions might be a good time to switch into more of an educational mode using a formal presentation than an interactive mode that depends on patient-to-patient feedback.

Outpatient Groups

Outpatient groups typically begin with a fixed number of patients who start together and continue until they are discharged. Such groups are called *closed* groups. Financial or agency requirements may limit the number of sessions to 12–20, and these groups are called *short-term time-limited* groups. If the group is ongoing, and one or two patients are discharged, then another one or two patients may be added. Two new additions are better than one in order to reduce the stress of being a single newcomer to a group. Such groups are called *slow-open* groups. As compared with their inpatient counterparts, members in outpatient groups are more stable and less acutely psychotic. Therefore, they can meet for longer sessions of 60 or even 90 minutes, although 45 minute sessions are still recommended for groups with more fragile patients or where teaching demands require post-group supervision to occur during the last 15 minutes of each hour. More patients can be accommodated than in inpatient groups. One therapist usually can manage outpatient groups, but if possible, two are better (see discussion on Cotherapy, below).

Issues involving two or three patients are similar to those discussed earlier for inpatient groups. Outpatient groups that typically have fewer than five patients per session are handicapped not only by cutting down the number of possible interactions, but also by creating an environment where members and therapists are overly concerned about patients not showing up in future sessions, to the point where they are afraid to challenge each other for fear that what they say may discourage people from coming. This creates a "too safe" group environment that hinders its therapeutic possibilities.

Formal Group Exercises

A typical session begins with either a silence or a therapist saying something like "What do you all want to talk about today?" Then he or she waits until a topic emerges that is congruent with the group goals. In this way, the patients feel responsible for the group, and someone who has a hot issue to discuss is given the freedom to mention it without being blocked by a predetermined agenda. Some therapists may want to do a "check-in" go-around, where each patient gives a progress report that summarizes how they were in the time interval between the previous and current sessions. Then, the group leader may ask the patients if any of the issues mentioned would be a good topic to begin with.

In the integrative model, there are three times when a formal exercise is used to begin a group: welcoming a new patient, saying goodbye to a discharged patient, or addressing a change in therapist.

Welcoming a New Patient

New patients should be screened by the leaders prior to entering the group. The screening process should first assess the accuracy of the patient's diagnosis and confirm that he or she has psychotic symptoms and relationship problems to work on. Then the leader describes the group's goals and format to make sure that the patient wants to become a member. Patients who agree then are scheduled to start at the next session. The continuing group patients need to have been told that a new patient is likely to start. At the first session, the following routine occurs:

> Vignette 4.11. The new patient first is introduced, then the leader conducts a go-around where everyone introduces themselves. The leader then states that the new person has been told that this is a group for people with nervous breakdowns, that it is meant to be a safe experience where people share ways to cope with their problems, and that discussions focus on issues such as hearing voices, feeling suspicious, being confused, or having problems relating with other people. Then the new patient is asked which of these problems he or she has. The therapist knows from the pre-group interview that at least one of these currently is a problem. If the patient denies any of them, the therapist reminds him or her that he mentioned one of them in the interview. Gentle prodding then continues that encourages the new patient to address the relevancy of all four targeted areas to him- or herself. When the new member is finished, the therapist says something like: "Well, you are not alone with these problems. Can someone else relate to them?" This takes the pressure off the new member, begins the process of encouraging group members to interact, and identifies one of the targeted areas as the topic to begin the session.

In this way, the new patient is encouraged to talk within the first few minutes of the group session, is helped to see that he or she is not alone with psychotic or interpersonal problems, and that discussions focus on these issues.

Saying Goodbye to a Discharged Patient

If possible, the group members are forewarned about an imminent discharge in previous sessions. During a member's last session, the leader makes the discharge the primary topic to start with:

> Vignette 4.12. The therapist states that this is the discharged patient's last session and asks him or her about the discharge plan and what he or she got out of the group experiences. The therapist then says a few words about progress the patient has made and invites the other members to do the same. An attempt is made to be upbeat and positive. Following this exercise, which should take around five to ten minutes, the therapist asks the group members what they want to talk about today, or, if a new member is also beginning, he or she is introduced according to the exercise described in Vignette 4.11.

Group members like to hear about discharge plans for a departing member and a recognition that the group was useful. Similarly, a patient who is leaving likes to hear from the leaders and the other group members of ways he or she has improved as a kind of graduation present before final goodbyes and well-wishes are made.

Addressing a Change in Therapist

A coleader who is planning to leave (either a staff member or a trainee) should announce his or her leaving and the departure date in the preceding session or two in inpatient groups or at least a month prior to leaving in outpatient groups. Patients then are asked for comments, if any, about the departure. On the day of departure, one of the leaders should announce the departure at the beginning of the session, and the following exercise should occur:

> Vignette 4.13. The departing therapist should say where he or she is going and any feelings about leaving the group. After this is done, the coleader can likewise say some words, to the effect that he or she will miss the departing therapist and wishes him or her well for the future. Then patients are asked to comment on their feelings regarding the departing therapist. Since it is useful for all patients to express their feelings about this important event, a go-around may be necessary in order to hear from everyone. This exercise should take around five to ten minutes. Then the departing patient exercise or the new patient exercise should occur if appropriate, or the patients are asked what they want to discuss for the day.

Departing therapists are a major event in the life of a therapy group, and the event often brings about feelings of abandonment or loss. Similarly, a new therapist introduced in the following group session is sometimes greeted with anger or a comparison with his or her previous counterpart. If such feelings occur, they should be labeled and discussed during the session.

Adjusting the Group Goals

As alluded to before, the two major treatment goals of integrative groups are dealing with psychotic symptoms and improving relationships The cognitive status of psychotic people varies, sometimes from session to session, so repetition of the group goals, member names, and major therapeutic elements are done frequently. But especially after four to six months, other issues emerge as well, such as the despair of having a chronic mental disease, the sequelae of societal stigma that may turn into self-stigma, the general mistrusting of others based on years of social isolation or maladaptive interactions, and memories of psychological problems based on early life traumatic events. How and when such issues are discussed depends on the state of the group.

Open Groups on Acute Care Inpatient Units

Table 4.6 summarizes how the group goals may be modified in different kinds of integrative groups. For open inpatient groups on acute care units, patients usually are very disturbed and enter into or are discharged from the group with great frequency. Learning that there is hope for them to be stable enough to be discharged and that they are not alone with their problems are very important therapeutic factors in the group. Beginnings can be made in ways to test reality and cope with hallucinations and delusions. There usually is not enough time to focus on relationship issues except for how their psychotic symptoms impact others (e.g., "Other people don't hear voices, so if you don't want to stick out on the bus, don't talk openly to yourself"). If patients hallucinate in the room, then this can become grist for the mill, as was described in Vignette 4.6.

With delusions, if a therapist tries too hard to challenge their reality, he or she may become incorporated into the delusion (e.g., become part of the secret society that is trying to hurt the patient). When a patient resists exploring the reality of psychotic productions, especially a delusion, it will be more helpful and less anxiety-producing to exit the topic, saying something like: "It sounds like you don't want to talk about this right now. Just keep in mind what I said and perhaps we can continue this discussion another time." Alternatively, more creative strategies may be

Table 4.6 Effects of setting and group developmental history on group goals

Setting/history	Effect on group goals
Open groups on acute care inpatient units	Main focus: testing reality and coping with current psychotic symptoms
	Interpersonal problems are discussed from the perspective of being related to psychotic symptoms
Newly formed outpatient groups, or closed short-term outpatient groups	Coping with psychotic symptoms and improving interpersonal relationships are discussed equally
	Good time to incorporate psychoeducational and CBT presentations in the discussion (e.g., A–B–C and vulnerability-stress models)
Later sessions of long-term groups (inpatient or outpatient)	Coping with psychotic symptoms are discussed less often than improving interpersonal relationships
	Long-standing problems and maladaptive patterns of relating are discussed with reference to their impact on current functioning (typically, after four–six months)

indicated to minimize anxiety and deal with the situation diplomatically, as the following vignette shows:

> Vignette 4.14. In an acute care inpatient group, new patient N began to describe his religious belief that he was Christ. Another new patient who was admitted a few days earlier, with the same belief about himself, became agitated, clenched his fists, and blurted out that he was Christ. Patient N then anxiously clarified that he was the "Servant of Man." The group leader, becoming concerned that both might escalate into a physical confrontation or regress into more psychosis, diplomatically asked N if being the "Servant of Man" was like being an Apostle, and after a moment he said yes, The other patient unclenched his fists, and both seemed to relax. This diplomatic solution allowed both patients to continue with their special grandiose delusion, one being Christ and the other an Apostle, and it decreased the tension in the room. Exploring these delusions would be put off to another day when both patients were more medicated and open to such a discussion.

Sometimes, creative strategies may lead to a successful challenge of a delusion:

> Vignette 4.15. In an acute inpatient group, which was conducted in a room outside of a locked unit, patient O repeatedly kept referring to his belief that the ward was a scary place based on posted messages that he was going to be killed. The leader asked the other patients if they knew what he was talking about. None of them did. So the therapist said: "Let's go look." He led all the patients out of the group room and onto the unit, where in the large day room there was a sign posted that was drawn by another patient. O said this was the indicator that he would be harmed on the unit. It showed an exploding nuclear reactor, with a skull and crossbones drawn below, and the written message at the top saying: "This could happen to you!" The therapist then led the patients back to the group room and asked the members to tell O what they thought of the sign. All of them said that it was an anti-nuclear power poster and had nothing to do with O. The therapist asked O if he believed this could be true, and he said: "Well, maybe so." Although the patient acknowledged some relaxation of his distorted belief about the unit, further discussion of the delusion was left for a later day.

One could argue about the advisability of displaying such a poster on a locked psychiatric unit, even though it was meant to encourage patient art. But the fact was that it was disturbing to a schizophrenic patient with persecutory delusions. Note, however, that he started the group session with a firm and fixed delusion, but that by the end of the session, he was beginning to challenge its reality. This slight change in emphasis was important for him in future discussions.

Newly Formed or Short-Term Outpatient Groups

As shown in Table 4.6, in newly formed outpatient groups, or in groups designed to be closed and short-term, the focus of the group varies between ways to test reality and cope with psychotic symptoms, and discussions of improving interpersonal relationships. Which goal is dealt with on a given day depends on what the patients or the leaders want to talk about. Typically, during these sessions, the therapist will begin with either no comment or a comment like: "What do you want to talk about today?" Topics unrelated to the group goals (like the weather or the fate of a local sports team or a favorite restaurant) can be ignored or passed over quickly by saying: "That's interesting, but it isn't the kind of thing we should take time to discuss here. What else?" When an appropriate topic is identified, the therapist tries to encourage the patients to give each other feedback in the here-and-now. Occasionally, the group leader will need to coach the patients to direct feedback to each other or to look at each other when they speak.

Early in the life of the group is a good time for the therapist to incorporate some psychoeducational or CBT material (such as white board diagrams of the A–B–C or vulnerability-stress models) into the discussion. Most discussions in early sessions relate to reality testing and coping with psychotic symptoms, or the anxiety that results from interacting with other people, so some degree of structured presentation can be useful to help them orient their thinking.

Long-Term Groups

Early in the life of a long-term group, the members have had plenty of opportunity to discuss topics related to coping with psychosis and improving interpersonal skills in their current life. After some four to six months, however, many patients are ready to take a look at long-standing problems (e.g., chronic distrust of people, distortions of the world based on idiosyncratic upbringing) and the sequelae of maladaptive or inexperienced patterns of relating (e.g., loaning money without promise of repayment, naiveté in bonding with others). By addressing such issues, they gain insight into how their current problems developed over time, which allows them to explore better ways of coping and interacting with others. Since some later sessions may deal with these non-psychotic topics, they may resemble discussions with a group of patients with depression or personality problems. But therapists must be cautious to keep anxiety and the direct expression of unpleasant affects in the here-and-now to a minimum in order to prevent regression and exacerbation of psychotic symptoms.

For some patients, the goals for success are modest. The leader must realize this and be content with whatever progress occurs. As an example:

> Vignette 4.16. During an outpatient group session, P, a 20-something paranoid schizophrenic man who had never had a date, volunteered that he was attracted to a woman in his sheltered workshop. Q, an older schizoaffective woman who had been acting very maternal toward P in the group, energetically gave him advice about how he should approach the young woman and things he could say to break the ice. The therapist supported some of these ideas and suggested that P try them out during the next week as homework. At the next session, P came in beaming, announcing that he had asked the woman to have coffee with him. She said yes, and he bought her a cup of coffee from a coffee machine. They chatted briefly and then went back to the workshop. P received much positive feedback from the other members of the group, including a joyous Q who obviously was happy with the success of her protégé.

This coffee date was a modest activity but a major event in P's life, and both he and Q shared in the success. For a withdrawn patient like P, it was a big step forward.

Discussion Topics

Topics discussed in integrative groups should be congruent with the group goals. If an irrelevant topic is brought up, the therapist ignores it, or passes over it, or says that the topic is not consistent with "what we talk about here." If the topic is relevant, the therapist perks up, asks questions, and may do a go-around to see how much interest in the topic there is among the group members in attendance. On occasion, an irrelevant topic, such as the success of a local baseball team or issues involving newsworthy events, may be allowed to continue, provided that they are safe topics, most of the members can relate to them, and the members spontaneously interact with good eye contact (which fulfils one of the group goals: relating with others in the here-and-now). Specific relevant topics depend on the setting and stage of the groups.

Early Groups

Some examples of discussion topics discussed during the group are shown in Table 4.7. Early in the life of the group, especially with acute patients, psychotic symptoms and ways to cope with them dominate the discussions. Ways of sensing what is real and strategies of testing reality

Table 4.7 Examples of discussion topics

Groups with acute patients or early in the life of the group

Improving reality sense and sharing strategies of testing reality (asking others, analyzing experiences logically, etc.)

Hallucinations (auditory, visual, tactile, etc.)

Delusions (persecutory, grandiose, jealousy, etc.)

Schneiderian first-rank symptoms (thought insertion, thought broadcasting, etc.)

Disorganized thinking (loose associations, tangential associations, flight of ideas, etc.)

Poor relationships with other (meeting people, maintaining relationships)

Safe emotions resulting from the illness (depression, hopelessness, etc.)

Groups with stable patients or late in the life of the group (typically after four to six months)

Above issues that are still unresolved

Difficult upbringing (absent or distant parent, substance abuse, sexual abuse, etc.)

Long-standing distorted schemas and beliefs about the world

Quality of attachments to parental figures and subsequent individuals

Long-standing distrust of other people

Naiveté in relationships (e.g., loaning money with no hope of repayment)

Despair over having a chronic illness

Social stigma toward psychosis and resulting self-stigma

Co-existing substance abuse

Topics that produce anxiety (anger over actions of people, sexual identity issues)—use caution to avoid decompensation

---

and coping with hallucinations and delusions (including those mentioned as Schneiderian first-rank symptoms—see Chapter 1) are uppermost in patients' minds. In fact, these issues often are demonstrated in the here-and-now of the group, such as when a patient hallucinates in the room or expresses a delusion about the ward staff. This is "manna from heaven," in that the therapist can explore the reality and phenomenology of the symptoms in real time in front of all the group members. Ways of coping can be discussed, with the other patients giving advice to the psychotic patient in a most visible and direct way. There is no second-guessing or memory distortions—what the group observes is what is happening. Loose associations also can be observed, and the therapist can address these directly:

> Vignette 4.17. In a new outpatient group, R was asked to describe his symptoms. He started out with a clear description, but gradually he drifted off into other topics. The therapist asked the other patients if they could follow what R was saying. Most said no. The therapist then observed that R was drifting off the topic and commented about how that makes communication difficult. He asked R

if he could understand this. R said yes. The therapist then asked him if in the future when he started to drift off, would it be OK for the therapist to interrupt and ask R to finish talking so that others could respond to his first point? He agreed, and this strategy was followed. Over time, R learned to self-regulate better and stop talking when he made one point. Whenever he did this, the group leader would positively reinforce his behavior with a compliment.

Disorganized thinking is best dealt with directly in the here-and-now of the sessions, rather than historically in the there-and-then, because it is a speech process issue rather than a content issue. As such, it is better observed than described.

Some relationship issues also can be discussed during early group sessions, but these relate primarily to the sequelae of psychotic symptoms: their impact on other people (both in and out of the group) and ways of behaving to avoid sticking out (e.g., while riding a bus). Emotions such as depression and hopelessness also can be discussed. Psychotic patients live in a despairing psychic world, and seeing that they are not alone with their feelings is often a paradoxically positive experience for them.

Later Groups

Unresolved issues related to symptoms and relationships should continue to be discussed throughout the life of the group. But new themes also may start to occur. Typically, after four to six months, discussions begin to deal more and more with issues related to upbringing and long-standing interpersonal issues. Many psychotic people are isolated and have not learned ways or relating with others during childhood and adolescence, so they often are naïve in their interactions and expectations. For example, they might loan strangers money and then wonder why they aren't repaid, or they are too trusting of others and don't know why people drop them or abuse them interpersonally. The quality of early attachments to parental figures and subsequent individuals may be explored, but cautiously so as not to provoke too much anxiety (see Attachment Theory in Chapter 2). Social stigma over having a serious, chronic mental illness contributes to the despair they feel and often is internalized as self-stigma. Many patients take sedatives to calm down or become addicted to alcohol and other drugs. The key in group is to address these various problems and relate them to the psychotic state. For example, many drugs (especially stimulants) make delusions worse, particularly in those patients who self-medicate rather than take prescribed medications. Feedback from patients who have had some success with medications and are otherwise abstinent may be helpful.

Emotions that produce anxiety or regression should be avoided. Care must be taken with themes related to sexual identity issues in the group.

For example, one patient in an inpatient group became visibly agitated when the topic turned to male–female relationships. It turned out that he had a fixed delusion that he was male above the waist and female below (despite being biologically male), and this confusion caused him great anxiety that was precipitated by the relatively benign discussion of dating.

Interpersonal anger also needs to be discussed with care. It is easy for therapists to be fooled, since the group is designed to be safe and conflict-avoidant, and patients who have been coming for a few months may appear to be better able to tolerate strong affects than they really are:

> Vignette 4.18. In a clinic outpatient group with schizophrenia spectrum patients that had been meeting for nearly six months, female patient S began angrily lambasting the only other female patient, T, for not supporting her more often. "After all," she said, "we are the only women here and must stick together." The four other male patients did not say much, and T looked visibly upset at being attacked. In the next session, T did not show up, and in fact she never returned to group. The men were unusually quiet, as if they were afraid that S would attack them as well. One of the two male group leaders commented on this behavior. He said that perhaps the last session was too intense for people and that it was important to keep the group safe and to confront issues, not people, in the group.

The two leaders allowed the angry feeling to be expressed, thinking that the patients could tolerate a little anger in the room. But this was not the case, and it resulted in a female patient dropping out and the male patients being traumatized for fear of being the next person attacked.

Coping Strategies

Examples of coping strategies are shown in Table 4.8. Sometimes, psychotic symptoms are made worse if a patient is either under- or over-stimulated by the environment. This is why it is useful for a patient to keep a record of what exacerbates or improves a symptom. It is also a good time in the group to do a presentation about the vulnerability-stress model (see Vignette 4.7) or the role of external stimulation in exacerbating symptoms using a "U" curve (see Vignette 4.9).

For patients whose symptoms are made worse by an over-stimulating environment (e.g., too many people, quarreling relatives, unpleasant news reports), the key is to reduce the stimulation. Leaving a toxic environment for a more soothing one is primary. Many physicians prescribe "prn" (i.e., "as needed") doses of medication for such times, and taking this dose may be helpful. Other ways to calm one's mind include counting to 10, reading a book, watching a relaxing TV show or movie, listening to

Table 4.8 Examples of coping strategies

If symptoms are made worse with high external stimulation
Leave the stressful situation
Take a prescribed prn ("as needed") dose of medication
Count to 10
Read a book
Watch a relaxing television show
See a relaxing, pleasant movie
Listen to quiet music
Walk in the woods or a park
Go to a museum
Take a warm bath
Meditate

If symptoms are made worse with low external stimulation
Go to a more stimulating environment
Take a prescribed prn dose of medication
Watch a stimulating television show, such as a sports event (avoid
   sensationalist news)
See an action movie that is not too arousing
Listen to stimulating music, like rock and roll
Walk in the city
Go to a museum
Go to a lecture
Do an activity with another person

Other coping strategies
Wait for the experience to stop on its own
Use logic to reality test the content of a hallucination or delusion
As a friend/relative/therapist about the reality of the experience
For auditory hallucinations, put on headphones or use ear plugs
Go into a secluded room and yell at the voices to go away
Go to church/synagogue/religious center or read the religion's Holy
   Scriptures
Develop a hobby, especially one that involves interacting with other people
   (e.g., chess club, quilting group, video games involving communications
   with other players)

quiet music, or going for a walk in a park or to a museum. For some people, a warm bath is helpful, and for meditators, mediation may be useful.

For patients whose symptoms are made worse by an under-stimulating environment (e.g., sitting in a quiet room listening to a dripping faucet that begins to sound like a "dripping" voice, noticing an upstairs neighbor's foot sounds and imagining that he or she is eavesdropping), going to a more stimulating environment and getting your mind onto something else is key. Examples include watching a stimulating TV show or listening to rock and roll music. A prn medication may help. Some people find it useful to take a walk in a city environment or go to a museum or a lecture. Action movies also may be helpful, if not too stimulating. Undergoing such activities with a friend or relative introduces another source of stimulation as well as providing an opportunity to interact with another person.

There are other coping strategies that people can use. Some chronic patients with long-standing experiences with psychosis can simply wait for the psychotic symptoms to abate on their own, or they use logical reasoning to test their reality. Asking a friend, relative, or therapist also is useful in reality testing. For auditory hallucinations, some patients find it useful to "block" the voices with headphones or ear plugs. Over the years, I have found that a significant number of patients get respite by going into a secluded room and yelling or swearing at the voices to go away. For religious patients, going to a church, synagogue, or another religious center is useful, as is reading Holy Scriptures. Developing a hobby also is helpful in getting one's mind off of hallucinations or delusions, and a hobby involving other people (such as a chess club or a quilting group) has the advantage of improving one's interpersonal life by being engaged in a common interest, where the interpersonal "ice is broken" by issues related to the hobby. Asking a friend to come along to an activity also has this advantage, and if the friend is another group member, then this sets up the possibility of a homework assignment, where the experiences of the interaction can be discussed in a follow-up session.

These and many other coping strategies may be suggested by one member to another, which is another reason why the leader of integrative groups encourages the patients to interact with each other. Even an idiosyncratic strategy may be useful for another patient to try. For example, following an integrative group discussion on ways to meet new people, a young patient volunteered that playing video games helped him to reduce his anxiety at meeting strangers. He said that in one video game he enjoys, several people play and communicate with each other via personal game-related avatars. These communications lead to discussions not only about the game and how people liked it, but also about more personal issues, which they can continue discussing after the game ends. The patient said that he was able to generalize what he learned from these experiences to real-life social contexts, such as parties or even day-to-day interpersonal interactions, and he experienced less anxiety and more confidence meeting new people as a result. Other members in the group who didn't play video games were intrigued by this person's experience and said they would give it a try.

Therapist Stance

The way a leader conducts any therapy group depends upon the needs of the patients and the goals of the group. With this in mind, I have

Table 4.9 Tips for the therapist

Be active and directive in keeping group members focused on the topic
Be clear, consistent, and concrete with interventions
Be supportive and diplomatic with comments to keep the group calm and safe
Be open and willing to give opinions and advice that further the discussion
Focus on the here-and-now rather than the there-and-then, unless you are
   trying to reduce anxiety
Encourage patient-to-patient rather than therapist-to-patient interactions,
   unless you are doing psychoeducation

---

compiled a list of tips for therapists leading integrative groups for psychotic patients, which is shown in Table 4.9. Many psychotic patients have trouble focusing their thoughts, so the leader needs to be active and directive in helping the group members stay on track while discussing issues related to the group goals. Since many psychotic patients also have problems with abstract ideas, therapeutic interventions need to be clear, consistent, and concrete. Note from the vignettes presented earlier that common English words are used instead of professional terms, such as "schizophrenic breakdown," "auditory hallucinations," or "persecutory delusions." Years ago, when I wrote my first book (Kanas, 1996), I reviewed many standard psychiatric textbooks and found that professional terms sometimes were used differently by different authors (e.g., the term "paranoid" varied from simple suspiciousness to ideas of reference to persecutory delusions to feelings of danger). I thought that if professionals differed in their use of professional terms, one can imagine how non-professionals might use them. Given also the observations that many psychotic patients are concrete in their thinking or have differing idiosyncratic interpretations of the same construct, it is important for group leaders to simplify their terms and make sure that patients understand the meanings that they intend.

Since many psychotic patients react poorly to anxiety and other strong emotions, the group leader should be mindful that the group environment remains safe and supportive. As discussed in Vignette 4.14, the therapist sometimes must be diplomatic in his or her comments, so that anger and escalating anxiety do not occur in the group. One tactic to achieve this is to make interventions less personal or to address the underlying issue in the there-and-then rather than the here-and-now (which is a much more emotional intervention). For example, if a patient becomes angry at another, the therapist might say something like: "You seem angry at John—what is it about what he said that makes you angry?" or "People sometimes make other people angry—who has made you angry like this in your past?" If this kind of diversion doesn't work, then simply say: "You know, anger at John seems to be making all of us uncomfortable, and we want the group to be safe for everyone. Let's all take a deep breath and find another issue to discuss today." Sometimes having the group members stand up and take a stretch break can reduce tension in the room (as well as wake up sleepy group members!).

As we shall see in Chapter 6, studies of the integrative group therapy model have shown it to be very similar in its process to other therapy groups across a number of variables, except that it scores high on research measures of "confrontation." What confrontation means here is not getting angry or rigidly challenging a patient. Rather, it is gently prompting him or her or the group-as-a-whole to discuss issues related to the group goals. If gentle reminders do not work, then more overt statements of the goals may need to be made, as was shown earlier in the section *Clinical illustration of a typical session.*

Sometimes, the group leader might offer an opinion or personal advice about an issue. This only should be done around issues that are not too personally revealing for the leader, and which advance the discussion rather than being said to make the leader feel better. Observations in the here-and-now are preferred to discussions of issues of the past in the there-and-then, and patient-to-patient feedback (with good eye contact) is preferred to therapist-to-patient interactions.

Cotherapy

In many therapy groups, particularly those with psychotic patients, having two leaders in the room has many advantages. First, if one is sick or on vacation, the other can still conduct the group without having to cancel a session. Second, if one leader is heavily engaged and making eye contact with a group member, the other can focus on the process or scan the room to look for nonverbal cues of distress or psychosis in other group members. Third, a cotherapy approach allows the two therapists to rehash issues that occurred after the session ends and plan for the next session. Fourth, treating psychotic patients can be a challenge, with goals that are modest in comparison to treating nonpsychotic patients, but techniques that are active and demanding. Two leaders can provide support and encouragement for each other, which helps prevent burnout. Fifth, it sometimes is helpful to get reality validation from another non-psychotic person in the room if the members are all agreeing on a viewpoint that has questionable validity or that presents an interesting philosophical premise that distracts the members from the group goals:

> Vignette 4.19. During a session of an inpatient group, one of the leaders was absent. Patient U began the session by stating his belief that there were several kinds of reality and that the reality expressed in the group and on the ward was no more valid than other realities.

The lone therapist asked the group members what they thought about this. To his surprise, the other members agreed with U and began a discussion of how many realities there were. The therapist found himself thinking about this issue as an interesting intellectual exercise. But then he realized that the discussion was becoming more philosophical that therapeutic. Because there was no cotherapist present, there was no other non-psychotic person in the room to validate the value of adhering to the present reality in order to function in this world. The group leader also was concerned that by being the only person taking an opposing position in the discussion, he might be seen by some of the patients as someone who wanted to persecute them. So the leader took a diplomatic position by saying that the issue being discussed certainly was interesting, but that it was not relevant to the goals of the group or to the patients' survival in the reality that was the ward, valid or not. He suggested another topic area, and the discussion moved to issues concerning relating better with other people in this reality.

Another advantage of having a cotherapist is to take care of an emergency involving a patient who decompensates or leaves the room:

Vignette 4.20. During a session of an outpatient group, V was happily talking about how his father was loaning him a computer and how the two of them would bond over using it to edit photographs. Patient W became distressed and bolted out of the room. One of the therapists went out after him and asked him what was going on to prompt his exit. He said that he was having a tough day and several times felt on the verge of a panic attack and having a crying episode, necessitating his taking a prn dose of medication before coming to group. He experienced similar panicky feelings during the group session, and this made him want to leave the room so that the other members wouldn't see him cry. He denied that the group had anything to do with these feelings, and he said that he was embarrassed to go back to the session. The therapist was planning to walk W to the access center for further evaluation, but fortuitously he saw W's primary therapist down the hall. He hailed her, and after explaining the situation, she said she was free to see him for an individual session. When asked, W said he planned to return to the group the following week.

The group therapist went back to the room and briefly told the group patients what had happened and that W said he would return to the group the following week. The coleader of the group said that during W's absence, she asked the remaining patients what they thought of his departure, and V said he felt guilty that something he had said prompted W to leave. The cotherapist assured V that what he said was appropriate for the group and that W's leaving was likely related to something he was going through himself.

The next week, W did in fact return. The therapist who had accompanied him out of the group the previous week commented that it was great for him to return, and he asked him if he wanted to say anything about the previous session. He said no, and the therapist said fine, but if he changed his mind, he should feel free to comment. The group moved on to other things. Later in the session, W volunteered that the issue of V's father last time made him feel sad about his own father's death, that it was not related to V himself, and that this was why he left. The therapist congratulated W for speaking up.

In situations where a group member suddenly leaves the room, one of the leaders should follow him out to assess his or her status. If necessary, a suicide/homicide evaluation might be needed (see Chapter 5), or the patient may need brief individual supportive therapy (like in Vignette 4.20), or medication. After the situation is stabilized, the therapist should return to the group room (hopefully with the patient) and inform everyone about what happened. In the meantime, the cotherapist's job is to assess how the remaining patients feel about the sudden departure, particularly probing for guilt feelings about causing the exit or anxiety about the event that might trigger regression or an exacerbation of psychotic symptoms.

In groups for nonpsychotic patients, where childhood experiences are part of the treatment, it is helpful to have a male–female cotherapy team to stimulate parental transferences. Because the integrative model for psychotic patients does not encourage uncovering and transference interpretations, it is not so important to have a male–female leadership team. However, some psychotic patients relate better to one sex or the other, and male–female coleaders can model opposite-sex interactions and viewpoints that may be helpful during gender-related discussions.

In cotherapy, it is important that the two leaders are seen as being equally valuable in the eyes of the patients, and they need to communicate clearly with each other during a session rehash to make sure that they are complimentary in their clinical approach. Training groups, where a student may function as a coleader, are by their nature unbalanced in terms of leadership experience, and this special cotherapy case will be discussed in Chapter 5.

Medications and the Integrative Group

Coleaders of integrative groups for psychotic patients do not need to be physicians. Although most of the group members are taking antipsychotic medications, these usually are prescribed by a medical doctor in a separate setting or clinic. Some patients receive medications from one of their group therapists if he or she is a psychiatrist, but this should be done during a different time (in some cases, the psychiatrist may see medication patients before or after the group session).

In contrast to special groups for non-psychotic bipolar patients (see Chapter 7), time rarely is taken during an integrative group therapy session for psychotic patients to discuss medication doses and side effects. These are best discussed in medication clinics or in individual meetings with physicians. In a similar manner, issues involving specific housing and occupational issues are best dealt with through social services. Since the integrative group is usually the only place where patients can openly discuss ways to cope with their psychotic experiences and improve their interpersonal interactions, precious time should be devoted to such issues. However, patients are allowed to discuss their feeling about having a chronic disorder that requires life-long medication treatment and the value of taking a prescribed prn dose of medication as a coping strategy for an exacerbation of their symptoms.

References

Drake, R.E. and Sederer, L.I. (1986) The adverse effects of intensive treatment of chronic schizophrenia. *Comprehensive Psychiatry*, 27(4), 313–326.

Francis, R. (2019) *On Conquering Schizophrenia: From the Desk of a Therapist and Survivor, with Purview on Metaphysics, Philosophy, and Theology.* Bloomington, IN: iUniverse Press.

Geczy, B. and Sultenfuss, J. (1995) Group psychotherapy on state hospital admission wards. *International Journal of Group Psychotherapy*, 45, 1–15.

Kanas, N. (1996) *Group Therapy for Schizophrenic Patients.* Washington, D.C.: American Psychiatric Press.

Kanas, N., Rogers, M., Kreth, E., Patterson, L. and Campbell, R. (1978) Psychiatric research in a military setting: Evolution of a study on inpatient group psychotherapy. *Military Medicine*, 143(8), 552–555.

Kanas, N., Rogers, M., Kreth, E., Patterson, L. and Campbell, R. (1980) The effectiveness of group psychotherapy during the first three weeks of hospitalization: A controlled study. *Journal of Nervous and Mental Disease*, 168, 487–492.

Kapur, R. (1993) Measuring the effects of group interpretations with the severely mentally ill. *Group Analysis*, 26, 411–432.

MacDonald, W.S., Blochberger, C.W. and Maynard, H.M. (1964) Group therapy: A comparison of patient-led and staff-led groups on an open hospital ward. *Psychiatric Quarterly*, 38(suppl.), 290–303.

Pattison, E.M., Brissenden, E. and Wohl, T. (1967) Assessing special effects of inpatient group psychotherapy. *International Journal of Group Psychotherapy*, 17, 283–297.

Pearson, M.J. and Burlingame, G.M. (2013) Interventions for schizophrenia: Integrative approaches to group therapy. *International Journal of Group Psychotherapy*, 63, 603–608.

Stone, W.N. (1996) *Group Psychotherapy for People with Chronic Mental Illness.* New York: Guilford Press.

Strassberg, D.S., Roback, H.B., Anchor, K.N. and Abramowitz, S.I. (1975) Self-disclosure in group therapy with schizophrenics. *Archives of General Psychiatry*, 32, 1259–1261.

Weiner, M.F. (1984) Outcome of psychoanalytically-oriented group psychotherapy. *Group*, 8(2), 3–12.

Yalom, I.D. (1983) *Inpatient Group Psychotherapy.* New York: Basic Books.

5 Clinical Issues of the Integrative Model
Special Topics

Introduction

In the previous chapter, basic clinical issues related to integrative therapy groups were discussed. These are the main issues that clinicians need to know to conduct such groups. In this chapter, I will consider special topics related to the therapists and patients who participate in integrative therapy groups, along with cost-effectiveness issues and the use of telepsychiatry.

Concurrent Group and Individual Therapy

Some patients may be seen in concurrent integrative group therapy as well as in individual therapy, which for psychotic patients generally is of the supportive type. Group therapy especially is indicated where a patient needs to improve his or her interpersonal interactions and where feedback from others with a similar condition might help the patient cope better and realize that he or she is not alone with problems. Supportive individual therapy especially is indicated where a patient is in a crisis and needs more attention or is acutely psychotic and very mistrustful or withdrawn.

In such concurrent situations, it is useful for different therapists to be involved in each modality (conjoint therapy). This allows for confidential information to be kept within each mode of treatment. But if this is the case, it is important for the therapists to communicate frequently with each other about a patient's status. At times, especially when resources are limited or in a crisis, the same therapist might see the patient in both modalities (combined therapy). Here, it is important for the therapist to keep boundaries clear and not reveal information received in individual treatment to other patients in group therapy, unless the patient gives permission.

Therapist Disclosure

As indicated in Chapter 2, group therapy patients typically rate advice received from the therapists low as compared with other therapeutic factors in groups. However, sometimes a therapist's advice is useful, such as during a psychoeducational or cognitive-behavioral therapy (CBT) session. But even in a general non-directive session, therapists may give advice that they feel clarifies or advances the discussion. This also applies to disclosing some personal information, which, in the integrative group therapy model, is allowable since transference issues usually are not interpreted in this approach. Although highly personal information, such as the therapist's sexual life or parental upbringing, rarely is appropriate to bring into the session, other information, such as a therapist's opinion about a clinical matter or personal experiences related to hypnagogic or hypnopompic hallucinations, may be helpful. In no case should a therapist use the group as psychotherapy to explore his or her own personal conflicts. Rather, for issues that are comfortable for the therapist to disclose and that illuminate or advance the discussion, describing personal experiences and giving advice may be of value to psychotic patients.

Difficult Patients

Disruptive Patients

A patient in the group who disrupts the conversation and prevents others from speaking may raise the anxiety level in the group. Usually, the cause of the disruption relates to psychotic symptoms (e.g., intruding voices, loose associations, uncontrolled outbursts). In such a case, pointing out the issue in the here-and-now may make the patient aware of his behavior and can even make the issue a productive discussion topic for all the patients:

> Vignette 5.1. In an outpatient integrative therapy group, patient X would occasionally laugh suddenly. The group leader asked X what was going on. He said that whenever the discussion led to an unpleasant topic, he would tell himself a joke or think an upbeat thought to cheer himself up. Then, he would laugh at his own thought. He said he couldn't help himself, and he wasn't laughing at anyone in the group. The therapist asked the other members what they thought of this, and most commented that it did bother them at first, but now that they understood what was going on, they felt that they could accept his occasional outbursts. The therapist commented to X that such unpredictable and uncontrollable behavior was a social handicap and must really be scary and inconvenient for him. X agreed, especially on buses where most people are quiet and are startled by his actions. This led to a general discussion about how other behaviors stemming from their psychosis, such as reacting to hallucinations or displaying bizarre movements from their disorder or from medication side effects, might draw unwanted attention in social situations. Like X, several patients had similar embarrassing experiences, and the group members discussed ways that they could use to hide or mask such actions in public.

X continued to laugh unexpectedly at times in the group, although the frequency decreased somewhat. Also, the group members did not take his actions personally and became tolerant of them, which made X more comfortable and trusting in the group.

When a disruption becomes so great as to interfere with the group process, the therapist may have to consider discharging the patient from the group. Recall that there are two "patients" in group therapy: the person speaking and the rest of the group members. When the actions of the former prevent the latter from benefiting from the sessions, then it may be time to transfer the offending person into individual treatment.

Monopolizing Patients

The same goes for monopolizing patients. Sometimes, continually talking or interrupting other patients is part of the psychotic process; but other times, it represents a personality style, with attention-seeking or passive-aggressive components. Often, identifying it and asking other patients to comment on how it affects them may be successful in curbing the monopolizing behavior. Alternatively, telling the patient that others in the group need to have their turn also may stop it. If these strategies don't work, then the patient may have to be transferred from the group into individual therapy. Like for patients with hallucinatory experiences or disorganized speech, patients who monopolize the group discussions need to be directable and able to control their behavior enough so as not to interfere with the therapy of the other patients.

Patients Requesting Frequent Bathroom Breaks

Sometimes, a patient will ask to leave the room to go to the bathroom. The therapist should ask him or her if there is something going on in the session that is disturbing or anxiety-producing, prompting his departure. If the patient convincingly says no, then he or she is excused, with the proviso that the patient comes back. After returning, the patient's return is acknowledged, and he or she is briefed on what has transpired in their absence. The patients are reminded to take care of bathroom needs and other disrupting activities (such as turning off their cell phones) before the group session starts in the future.

If, in a following session, the patient again requests to leave for the bathroom, he or she may be gently confronted upon returning about repeatedly leaving for this reason. This issue may become a topic for the group to discuss, especially if other patients begin requesting bathroom breaks or other departures from the session in order to prevent such departures from becoming disruptive group norms.

Suicidal/Homicidal Patients

Occasionally, patients in the integrative group will express suicidal or homicidal ideation.

Like with any group patient, where such ideation is reported, a moment of group time should be taken to assess the following: (1) presence of definite ideation, (2) intent to act, (3) definite plan of action, and (4) means to accomplish the deed (such as owning a weapon or having toxic medications or drugs available). With a psychotic patient, such ideation often takes the form of voices commanding him or her to hurt himself or others. Given the high risk of such a psychotic patient actually acting on these voices, the group leader should take such experiences seriously, particularly if the patient says that the voices are new or expresses concern about losing control and doing what they command. If the patient cannot be assessed properly in the group, then the therapist should see the patient individually after the group and do a more formal evaluation. Any psychotic patient who has definite ideation or command hallucinations of harming himself or others, who has a plan or expresses fears of giving in to the impulses, and who does not have a solid support system to monitor his behavior when he leaves the group should be considered for admission to the hospital.

For non-suicidal patients who experience despair and loneliness related to their illness, talking about such feelings in the group often results in a positive outcome, not only for a given patient but for the other group members as well who may feel the same way:

> Vignette 5.2. In an inpatient group, Y, a relatively stable patient with schizophrenia who was about to be discharged, began talking about his loneliness. He described being withdrawn from people for nearly a decade since his first breakdown. He denied suicidality but acknowledged feelings of despair over his condition. In response, another patient said that he too felt lonely growing up in a large family. The therapist commented that the two of them had much in common, and he suggested that perhaps they could continue a social relationship after both were discharged. They seemed open to this suggestion. When the session ended and the two of them walked out of the room, the other patient gently patted Y on the shoulder, a non-verbal indicator of support and commonality that the two men felt for each other.

These two patients learned that they were not alone in their feelings about their psychotic condition, and this allowed them to bond and experience less isolation and despair as a result of the group discussion.

Patients with Negative Symptoms

In the integrative model, all patients are invited to speak at some point during the session. If a patient really doesn't want to talk, then he or she may be left with comments such as:

> Maybe later you will feel like talking, and if so, feel free to jump in. If not, then maybe next session you will be more inclined to talk. But for now, you can participate by just listening to what is being said.

Patients with prominent negative symptoms (as well as extremely paranoid patients) are especially unresponsive in a group setting. The therapist should address such a patient at least once in every session and comment on how hard it must be for them to come out of his or her shell. Every opportunity should be given to encourage these patients to participate when ready.

Licensed social worker Robert Francis has described the method he uses to cope with the negative symptoms of his schizophrenic disorder:

> For me, regular physical and cognitive activity are part of my coping strategy. I often have to will myself to engage in activity, but once engaged in my habitual activities, amotivation as a symptom generally loses its causal efficacy. At this point, amotivation is low on my list of problem symptoms due in part to my primary strategy to always stay involved, active, and "in the game" as best I can regardless of current symptoms.
>
> (Francis, 2019, p. 53)

Based on Francis's experience, an approach for helping psychotic patients with negative symptoms is to give them homework assignments. For example, he or she may be given a simple exercise in the group, such as to role-play asking someone on the bus about the next stop, then practice doing this action outside of the group on a real bus and reporting back the results in the next session. Another homework assignment might be to read about a potential new hobby and report back to the group what was learned, then discussing ways that he or she can seek out other people interested in this hobby. Forcing oneself to be active in a task that might be pleasurable helps to conquer the amotivational aspect of psychosis.

Sometimes, a patient who is quiet and withdrawn in the group absorbs more than one might think:

> Vignette 5.3. In an inpatient group, a patient with prominent negative symptoms was encouraged to speak several times in every session, but his comments were nonexistent or minimal each time, such as a simple "yes" or "no." When asked about this, he said he preferred not to speak. However, he seemed to be alert and made eye contact with

other group members who were speaking. When it came time for him to be discharged, the therapist asked him what he had gotten out of the group, thinking that again his comments would be minimal. To everyone's surprise, he spoke up, saying that he learned that he was not alone with his problems, and that seeing other people getting better gave him hope that he too would become well enough to be discharged. He also referred to specific topics that had been discussed in the group, and he said that he had learned ways of coping with his problems from the experiences of other group members. He thanked the therapist and the patients for helping him.

Although it is easy to see positive symptoms change for the better in group patients, even those with negative symptoms can benefit from their group experience, albeit in a more passive and subtle manner.

Medication Compliance

As we shall see in Chapter 8, compliance with medication is a problem for patients with bipolar disorder, which is especially tragic since taking mood stabilizing medications greatly improves the course of this illness. Patients with schizophrenia spectrum disorders similarly have compliance issues; but for them, medications sometimes are wrapped up in delusional thinking about putting poison or strange substances into their bodies. Also, many patients do not like the side effects of antipsychotic medications and prefer to look at alternatives to lessen anxiety and deal with psychotic symptoms, such as meditation and religious practice. Usually in my integrative groups, there is at least one patient who is medication-resistant. I try to get the other patients to speak about the benefits of properly prescribed medications, but this often is not successful. Refusal to take medications is not a contraindication to being admitted to my integrative groups, provided that the patient is directable and can participate without being too much of a distraction to the other patients. And after all, the focus of my group model is to look at non-medication strategies of coping with psychosis.

Francis has this to say about the role of medications in his disorder:

> I must assert the importance of medication over the course of my schizophrenia. Without meds, psychosis prevails…Without medication, my mind shatters and my life scatters. Lucid becomes anomaly and horror the norm…medication and its efficacies is a primary protective factor.
>
> (Francis, 2019, p. 130)

He goes on to say that insight and the supportive relationship of his family are two other primary protective factors.

Philosophy and Religion

As noted in the previous chapter, an important goal of the integrative group model is to help patients learn to sense and to test reality. But what exactly is reality? Francis (2019) has discussed some of the philosophical implications of this question. Patients in the integrative group also like to discuss this issue, and it is important not to use up too much group time philosophizing about the nature of reality versus helping patients learn ways of dealing with the shared reality of people around them, as was illustrated in Vignette 4.19 in the last chapter.

Psychotic people have a great interest in such philosophical discussions, probably because the world they live in is confusing, and they find themselves thinking ideas that non-psychotic people (other than philosophers!) rarely consider. Francis echoes this dilemma:

> The concepts of my mind are at times synchronized with mutually shared reality, but additionally, are also at times not in sync with said reality and are characteristic of psychotic thought. In this manner, my personal conceptual reality accounts for both the rational and psychotic, and therefore the whole to my experience remains integral.
>
> (Francis, 2019, p. 89)

The best strategy in the group is to avoid philosophical excursions and to discuss practical issues of reality that will best serve the needs of the patients.

Religion is another issue that many psychotic patients find rewarding. In fact, religious patients often get great solace from their religion and find that attending church or synagogue or other religious gatherings and reading Holy Scriptures can help them cope with frightening delusions and hallucinations. I encourage such patients to practice their religion, not only for the belief aspect but also for the socialization aspect of being around other like-minded people with whom they can interact and gain comfort.

In some cases, religion becomes incorporated into a positive psychotic experience, as the following excerpts from Francis's book illustrate:

> One positive psychotic experience I had was an episode in my late twenties about five years into the illness. I found myself in a perceived literal dialogue with God, not aloud but in my mind, and I perceived the dialogue as real. I had no doubts about the experience. I was immersed in the belief. It was not a prayerful monologue but rather a one-to-one conversational communion.
>
> (Francis, 2019, p. 69)

Regarding the content of the conversation, he goes on to say:

> I felt so entirely persecuted by the world that my only perceived salvation during this time of hopelessness and darkness was an appeal

to God. Then, while I was occupied in prayer and petition and from the eye of my contemplation, God spoke. And upon word one, my despair was abruptly vanquished then followed by the further miraculous. Light permeated my being. A sublimity filled the depths of my pores...God explained to me my suffering and it made complete sense. God explained to me that historically others too have been persecuted but that in his wisdom it had purpose and meaning and that was benevolent.

(Francis, 2019, p. 70)

God went on to explain that he would "show me heaven on Earth," Francis states, and he explained nature and creation. Then the conversation turned humorous:

God joked, and it was all too funny. I ultimately made it to my destination, that being the pizza shop, and I grabbed a slice and sat at the booth. Then after a few more humorous comments by God, the experience abruptly ended.

(Francis, 2019, p. 71)

This experience helped Francis feel better during a period of time that he felt persecuted and in despair, and the experience and conversation were real to him. But such religious experiences can have a downside as well:

I think the most difficult persecutory delusional content I have endured is the recurrent episode of being rejected by all of humanity along with being rejected by God, as well. For where else is one to turn? All has been negated, and nothing is seemingly left as refuge.

(Francis, 2019, p. 43)

For most religious psychotic patients, their religion is a positive influence that functions as a useful coping strategy to help them with hallucinations and negative feelings.

Training and Supervision

The integrative model is easy to teach to mental health trainees, such as interns or residents in psychiatry, psychology, psychiatric social work, psychiatric nursing (especially nurse practitioners), and allied specialties. It is best to give the students handouts of the treatment approach and to meet with them at least once prior to their beginning the group in order to orient them to the model. Some experience in psychotherapy (individual, family, or group) is useful, as is prior involvement with psychotic patients.

Inexperienced students participating in the group often begin as co-leaders with more experienced therapists. The problem here is the relative inequality of experience, and patients pick this up right away. But it is not an insurmountable problem, since many patients feel proud that they are helping to train new group therapists, and they value the input from a younger person with a different perspective than the senior therapist.

At the beginning, the trainee is reluctant to participate, choosing to observe for a while. I tell students that when you begin to think about a topic or issue just before I say it, it means that you are becoming sensitive to the group process. I encourage students to say something in the group as soon as possible, even if it is just a simple "hello" or supportive comment affirming the validity of what the patient is saying. I give the student three or four sessions to break in, then encourage them in our after-group supervisory sessions to take the plunge during the next session, or even to begin the session themselves with a simple "let's get started" or "does anyone have anything to talk about today?"

Cultural Issues

Therapy groups based on the integrative model have successfully been conducted in special culture-sensitive units in the United States consisting of African-Americans, Asian immigrants, and Asian-Americans. They also have been conducted abroad, such as in an inpatient psychiatric unit in Russia (Kanas, 1991) and in England. Articles describing this model have been translated into Japanese (Kanas, 1992a, b). Clinical and empirical findings have supported this model in such settings, and local staff and trainees were trained in the clinical approach in a relatively brief period of time.

Although signs and symptoms of schizophrenia spectrum disorders tend to be similar around the world, specific cultural factors sometime need to be considered in integrative therapy groups. At times, these dominate the session:

> Vignette 5.4. At the San Francisco General Hospital, culture-sensitive units were set up oriented around the special needs of patients from different minority groups in the city. One such unit focused on African-Americans. During one integrative group session, the group began by discussing suspicious thoughts and how to test the reality of the suspicion. Z, a patient with paranoid schizophrenia, blurted out that he could not trust any white people, and he alluded to the presence of a white conspiracy permeating the country. When one of the therapists (an African-American nurse) challenged the generality of this statement, other patients began to defend Z. The topic then switched to social issues involving discrimination. The group leaders acknowledged that discrimination occurred and tried to reframe the conversation in terms of reality testing and patient symptoms. The group members could not make this transition, and the rest of the session became a general discussion of discrimination in American society.

On this unit, issues of discrimination were discussed frequently in a variety of settings. This fusing of emotional social issues with issues related to psychosis sometimes was difficult to separate, like in this session. Rather than persist, the therapists chose to let the patients discuss discrimination, since they were interacting with one another with good eye contact and supported each other for what they were saying. Delusional issues related to persecutory beliefs were addressed in a later session.

In another unit at the same hospital for Asian immigrants and Asian-Americans, an integrative group was begun. Because several Asian cultural groups were represented, the group was conducted in English, which unfortunately eliminated some immigrants who didn't speak this language. Other potential patients refused to attend because of a fear of losing "face" by admitting their problems in front of other people. To assure that there were enough members to compose a group, a few patients were admitted from an adjoining ward. Thus, a successful group was formed, which despite the cultural heterogeneity was diagnostically homogeneous in terms of schizophrenia spectrum disorder. Unlike the black-focus group mentioned above, this group tended to minimize cultural issues and focused on ways of dealing with psychosis.

During a sabbatical in St. Petersburg, Russia (then called Leningrad, Soviet Union), I set up an integrative group on a unit at a psychiatric teaching hospital. The group was conducted in the Russian language and consisted of four female schizophrenic patients and two therapists (a female staff clinical psychologist and a male psychiatric resident). I trained the therapists in the model and supervised the group from outside the group circle with the help of an English-speaking translator by my side. There was some concern that Russian patients, who were brought up in the somewhat restricted Soviet society, would be more private and guarded than their American counterparts, and that the more formal doctor–patient relationship in the Soviet Union might restrict the give and take typically found in Western groups. Indeed, in the first session, the therapists were quite deferential to the patients, hesitating to probe into personal matters and sometimes asking permission to inquire about their feelings. The patients tended to be quiet and minimally responsive to the therapists, and they did not interact much with each other. During the supervision following this session, I suggested that the therapists be more active and directly ask the patients if as a result of their psychiatric problems they heard voices, felt suspicious, experienced confused thoughts, or had problems relating with others. I also described some techniques the group leaders could use to get the patients to interact with one another during the sessions.

The next session began much like the first. However, mid-way, the staff psychology therapist asked one of the patients if she heard voices. She said "yes" and indicated that it was embarrassing for her to admit this in front of other people. When the therapist invited the other members to comment, all responded supportively and shared their own psychotic symptoms and the problems they caused during the remainder of the session. After the session, the psychologist therapist expressed surprise at how much the patients revealed and how readily they responded to this gentle prompting. In subsequent sessions, the therapists were much more direct and active, with good results.

Although the reluctance of the therapists to confront their patients might have been due to their inexperience with the treatment method and the fact that I was observing them, it also seemed to reflect attitudes related to Soviet society, where the therapist–patient relationship was more formal and where it might be dangerous to reveal too much to strangers. However, when the therapists became more active and clearly indicated that what was being asked pertained to their symptoms, the patients responded by opening up, and the group began to resemble an integrative group composed of American schizophrenia spectrum patients.

Similarly, cultural factors seemed to have been transcended in an inpatient integrative group at a general hospital outside London, UK. Although the patients were British subjects, they were quite diverse culturally. For example, of the 20 patients who participated in 10 sessions of an integrative group, 12 were male; there were 10 black, 8 white, and 2 Asian patients; and several were born in different countries. In addition, to have enough psychotic patients to form a group, patients were recruited from two separate units, with one coleader from each unit. Despite this diversity, the group scored highly on a measure of cohesion, and over three-quarters of the discussion topics were related to coping with psychotic experiences and interacting better with other people (see Chapter 6 for additional research findings). Thus, if the therapists focus on problems related to psychosis, the group members still will be able to bond together around common needs despite cultural and demographic diversity.

Cost-Effectiveness of Integrative Groups

In the next chapter, research findings will be presented that support the effectiveness of the integrative approach for psychotic patients. As we shall see, patients participating in integrative groups experience reductions in symptoms and social anxiety, and they report improvement in coping with psychotic symptoms and relating with other people after the group ends. More than half of the psychotic patients completing a short-term, time-limited integrative group elect to participate in a similar group experience within two years. Attendance rates typically are in the 80%–90% range, and outpatient dropout rates generally are less than 20%.

Health insurance claim data and meta-analyses of controlled studies have converged to show that psychotherapy (including group therapy) provides a cost-offset in terms of reducing subsequent medical services (Mumford et al., 1984). In general, group therapy is as useful as individual therapy and also is more efficient in terms of the number of patients treated (Toseland and Siporin, 1986). Patients who participate in inpatient groups are more likely to participate in outpatient groups (Yalom, 1983). Outpatient therapy groups for patients with schizophrenia may result in lower rehospitalization rates and less time spent in the hospital during subsequent readmissions (Alden et al., 1979; Battegay and von Marschall, 1978; Shattan et al., 1966).

Less clinician time is spent in group therapy than in individual therapy. For example, in a group of eight patients being seen for an hour, the staff–patient ratio is 2:8 where cotherapy is used, and 1:8 where there is just one leader; the same eight patients would require eight individual therapy hours. In addition, the integrative model encourages patients to learn ways of relating better with other people and includes practice in interacting during the group sessions. This interpersonal focus is less well addressed in individual therapy. So in conclusion, integrative therapy groups are helpful and cost-effective for psychotic patients.

Telepsychiatry and Integrative Groups

The use of online telepsychiatry offers many challenges for group therapy. Only patients who can access Zoom or a similar platform on a personal device or a computer with a camera can participate. Since patients appear on a screen array, not in a group circle, they cannot make eye contact with each other. To remedy this, the leaders and members should state the name of the person to whom they are speaking, and the leaders can ask the patients to look at a person being addressed on their screens. Another challenge is that it is impossible to pick up non-verbal behavioral cues in areas of the body not shown on the screen. There sometimes are technical problems where a patient temporarily loses connection, but usually a simple phone call to the patient will help restore the connection. At times, there is a distraction in the patient's environment, such as a person or pet, and these intrusions need to be addressed by the leader.

When the COVID-19 virus pandemic hit the United States, most states, including California, imposed physical distancing. As a result, I decided to run an outpatient psychosis group based on the integrative model using the Zoom platform. Patients agreed to adhere to a written privacy and confidentiality form prior to entering the group. They also provided the phone number and location of where they would be during the sessions in case of an emergency that required first responder presence. At the time the proofs for this book were returned, there were five male and one female patients in the group, all with schizophrenia spectrum diagnoses. Two psychiatric nurse practitioner trainees and I were the coleaders. The group had met for 14 weekly sessions that lasted for 45 minutes each. New patients continue to be admitted, with the goal of six to eight attendees per session.

The group has been well-received. Attendance has been 91% of expected participation, and there have been no dropouts. The goals of the group have been addressed, and the discussions have been similar to previous in-person groups. Educational materials, such as diagrams of the A–B–C and vulnerability-stress models and the "U" curve external stimulation-symptom relationship, were prepared in advance and used in screen-sharing during appropriate sessions. Since many of the patients live alone or in restricted environments, the group provides an educational and supportive experience for them during the week. All in all, where in-person groups are not possible, telepsychiatry represents a viable alternative.

References

Alden, A.R., Weddington, W.W. Jr., Jacobson, C. and Gianturco, D.T. (1979) Group aftercare for chronic schizophrenia. *Journal of Clinical Psychiatry*, 40, 249–252.

Battegay R. and von Marschall, R. (1978) Results of long-term group psychotherapy with schizophrenics. *Comprehensive Psychiatry*, 19, 349–353.

Francis, R. (2019) *On Conquering Schizophrenia: From the Desk of a Therapist and Survivor, with Purview on Metaphysics, Philosophy, and Theology.* Bloomington, IN: iUniverse Press.

Kanas, N. (1991) Group therapy in Leningrad. *Group*, 15, 14–22.

Kanas, N. (1992a) Group therapy with schizophrenic patients: A short-term, homogeneous approach (translated in Japanese). *Journal of the Japan Association of Group Psychotherapy*, 8, 83–92.

Kanas, N. (1992b) Group therapy with schizophrenics: American and Japanese perspectives (in Japanese and English). *Journal of the Japan Association of Group Psychotherapy*, 8, 100–102.

Mumford, E., Schlesinger, H.J., Glass, G.V., Patrick, C. and Cuerdon, B.A. (1984) A new look at evidence about reduced cost of medical utilization following mental health treatment. *American Journal of Psychiatry*, 141, 1145–1158.

Shattan, S.P., Dcamp, L., Fujii, E., Fross, G.G. and Wolff, R.J. (1966) Group treatment of conditionally discharged patients in a mental health clinic. *American Journal of Psychiatry*, 122, 798–805.

Toseland, R.W. and Siporin, M. (1986) When to recommend group treatment: A review of the clinical and the research literature. *International Journal of Group Psychotherapy*, 36, 171–201.

Yalom, I.D. (1983) *Inpatient Group Psychotherapy.* New York: Basic Books.

6 Evaluation of the Integrative Model

Introduction

In Chapter 3, I presented a number of controlled studies, reviews, and meta-analyses that supported the value of the interpersonal, psychoeducational, and cognitive-behavioral (CBT) approaches to group therapy for psychotic patients. The psychoanalytic/psychodynamic approach also was supported, but weakly, and with a caution that if it emphasized too much anxiety-producing uncovering and affect expression, it could be harmful for some psychotic patients. All four of these approaches are represented in my integrative model; so in a sense, the studies in Chapter 3 provide some face validity to my approach.

My integrative model did not originate from any specific theory or approach. Rather, it developed empirically from a series of outcome and process studies that led to the final clinical model described in Chapters 4 and 5. I started conducting therapy groups for psychotic inpatients shortly after I arrived at the San Francisco Department of Veterans Affairs Medical Center (SFVA) in 1977. My colleagues and I evaluated the group's outcome and process empirically, then altered the approach, then studied it further, and so on. This chapter will review these studies, which are divided in terms of inpatient and outpatient settings. Most of the groups deal primarily with schizophrenia spectrum patients, although a few psychotic bipolar patients and patients with unspecified psychoses were included along the way.

Inpatient Studies

The earliest inpatient studies took place on a 30-bed acute care locked psychiatric unit at the SFVA (Kanas and Barr, 1983). The average length of stay on the unit was three weeks, although patients with schizophrenia tended to remain about five and a half weeks. The group based on the integrative model was homogeneously composed of psychotic patients, most of whom were men diagnosed with schizophrenia spectrum disorder. It met initially for one hour on a weekly basis, but it soon settled into 45-minute sessions that met three times per week. The approach was supportive, tended to mute strong affects, and focused on dealing with psychotic symptoms and improving interpersonal relationships rather than gaining insight or uncovering unconscious conflictual material. In polls of the unit staff, most felt that this group helped the patients become less fearful of and interact better with other patients and staff on the ward. Based on this input, we decided to formally study the outcome and process of this group.

In the first study (Kanas and Barr, 1982), 22 schizophrenia spectrum patients completed an integrative group therapy discharge questionnaire after participating in an average of nine group therapy sessions on the locked ward at the SFVA. On the questionnaire, the patients were first asked to assess how helpful the group had been for them overall, with ratings of "harmful," "neither helpful nor harmful," "somewhat helpful," and "very helpful." They then were asked to rate a series of 13 statements according to how important a factor each was in their treatment, with ratings of "not at all," "somewhat," or "very" important. Some of the statements were based on the then current version of the therapeutic factor system of Yalom (1975)—see Chapter 2. Other statements were added to reflect psychotic symptomatology. After completion, all of the ratings were given scores: "2" for very important, "1" for somewhat important, and "0" for not at all important. Based on the total scores, the 13 statements could be rank-ordered. Patients also were given space to write in responses to questions about what they liked most and least about the group, and to add other thoughts on ways to make the group experience better for future patients. The current version of the questionnaire is shown in Figure 6.1.

Overall, 95% of the respondents rated their group experience as being "very" or "somewhat" helpful. The "very" category was endorsed by significantly more subjects below the median age of 29.5 years and subjects with non-paranoid diagnoses.

The total points and ranking of the therapeutic factor questions are shown in Table 6.1. The patients valued the group more as a place to express feelings, learn ways of relating better with others, and cope with psychotic symptoms than as a place to gain insight in the causes of their problems or receive practical advice on their illness and its treatment. This ranking seems appropriate for a group of inpatients on an acute care psychiatric unit. In the write-in section, ten patients commented that it was a good place for them to talk, an additional four said that they liked the other group members, and another four said that there was nothing they liked least. No other trends were apparent.

A second inpatient study evaluated the group process using the Hill Interaction Matrix (Hill, 1961, 1965). This well-known process measure classifies groups in terms of the content being discussed and the manner in which the group works to help the members learn more about themselves. The four content categories are: topical areas, the group itself,

How <u>helpful</u> was this group overall (circle one rating):

    harmful   neither helpful nor harmful   somewhat helpful   very helpful

Rate the statements as to their <u>importance</u> for your treatment (circle one rating per statement):

The group allowed me a place to express my emotions.	not at all	somewhat	very
The group showed me that I am not the only one with problems.	not at all	somewhat	very
The group helped me become less suspicious of others.	not at all	somewhat	very
The group showed me that I can help other people.	not at all	somewhat	very
The group taught me how to relate better with people.	not at all	somewhat	very
The group helped me decide the difference between reality and my imagination.	not at all	somewhat	very
The group helped me cope better with my voices and/or visions	not at all	somewhat	very
The group helped me feel hopeful about my future.	not at all	somewhat	very
The group gave me insight into the causes of my pr oblems.	not at all	somewhat	very
The group gave me useful advice about the nature of my illness.	not at all	somewhat	very
The group gave me useful advice about medications.	not at all	somewhat	very
The group helped me learn to control some of my emotions.	not at all	somewhat	very
The group gave me useful advice about jobs, finances, or places to stay.	not at all	somewhat	very

What did you like <u>most</u> about the group?

What did you like <u>least</u> about the group?

How can I make this group <u>better</u> for future patients?

Figure 6.1 Integrative Group Outcome and Process Questionnaire.

personal issues, and relationships. The four work categories are: conventional, assertive, speculative, and confrontive. Each group session can be scored along these eight dimensions by the patients, the group leader, or an outside observer, and the scores can be compared to a normative sample of 50 therapy groups of patients who generally were non-psychotic or substance abusing. The two categories also can be placed in a 4 × 4 matrix to produce 16 content/work cells. There are important clinical ratios that can be calculated, such as the amount of contribution by the therapists versus the patient members. If this Th/M ratio is above 1.00, then this tells us that the therapist is relatively active in directing the group.

Table 6.1 Ranking of therapeutic factors in a short-term inpatient group (Kanas and Barr, 1982)

Therapeutic factor statement	Points	Rank
The group allowed me a place to express my emotions.	36	1
The group showed me that I am not the only one with problems.	34	2
The group helped me become less suspicious of others.	31	3
The group showed me that I can help other people.	27	4
The group taught me how to relate better with people.	26	5
The group helped me decide the difference between reality and my imagination.	24	6
The group helped me cope better with my voices and/or visions.	22	7
The group helped me feel hopeful about my future.	22	7
The group gave me insight into the causes of my problems.	21	9
The group gave me useful advice about the nature of my illness.	19	10
The group gave me useful advice about medications.	19	10
The group helped me learn to control some of my emotions.	18	12
The group gave me useful advice about jobs, finances, or places to stay.	15	13

Since we had access to a one-way mirror and nurses interested in being trained in the system, we used the 72-item version of the Hill Interaction Matrix called the HIM-G, whereby an outside observer did the scoring of each group session.

Kanas, Barr and Dossick (1985) studied seven triweekly sessions of an integrative group at the SFVA using a nurse evaluator trained in the HIM-G system to observe and score the sessions. Eleven different male inpatient patients with schizophrenia participated in the group during the study interval. The 45-minute sessions averaged five patients and two therapists trained in the integrative system. The second column in Table 6.2 shows the percentile scores for this group compared with the Hill normative sample. Note that the group fell into the non-significant range in seven of the dimensions, but it was at the 97th percentile in the Confrontive category. This category of work is "characterized by a penetration to the significant aspects of a discussion; and because of this penetration, these statements confront members with aspects of their behavior usually avoided" (Hill, 1961, p. 54). It is notable that this category is felt to be the highest level of group work in the Hill system, since groups high in this category engage in risk-taking and honesty in interacting, rather than fault-finding or attacking behavior (Hill, 1965). Furthermore, the Topic/Confrontive matrix cell scored at the 99th+ percentile. The Hill scoring manual says that ratings in this cell

are given to interaction in which discussions of pertinent topics about mental health or adjustment are synthesized or characterized

Table 6.2 HIM-G category percentile scores for integrative groups versus normative groups

Category	SFVA inpatients (Kanas, Barr and Dossick, 1985)	SFVA inpatients (Kanas and Smith, 1990)	SFVA outpt. repeaters (Kanas and Smith, 1990)
Content style			
Topic	75	68	70
Group	56	82	65
Personal	43	26	34
Relationship	49	58	60
Work style			
Conventional	34	48	52
Assertive	64	68	60
Speculative	35	14	13
Confrontive	97[a]	98[a]	98[a]

a Statistically significant.

in a penetrating and usually insightful fashion so that each member is personally confronted by the implications of the material being discussed.

(Hill, 1961, p. 55)

The only category where the Th/M ratio was above 1.00 was in the Confrontive category, suggesting that the therapists were active in encouraging the patients to discuss significant aspects of their illness. The therapists were active overall, commenting 10%–20% of the time during the sessions. Patients were engaged, failing to react to the therapists less than 1% of the time, and the group environment was safe, with group resistance occurring less than 1% of the time.

This study was replicated five years later on the same unit (but now with 28 beds) and different therapists, different patients, and a different rater (Kanas and Smith, 1990). Twelve consecutive triweekly 45-minte sessions consisting of 11 different male schizophrenia spectrum patients were evaluated, again with an average of five patients and two therapists per session. The third column of Table 6.2 shows similar results to the second column, with the Confrontive work style category again defining the uniqueness of the group (98th percentile) when compared to the normative sample. The Topic/Confrontive matrix cell again scored at the 99th+ percentile. The rank order of the 16 category X work matrix cells in the two studies was compared using the Spearman Rank-Order Correlation (rho), and the results showed a highly significant correlation (p < .01). Again, the therapists were active (26% of the total session time), especially in the Confrontive category (Th/M ratio = 1.22), and patients were minimally responsive and resistive only 1%–5% of the time.

Group process was evaluated in another SFVA inpatient study using a different measure: the short form of the Group Climate Questionnaire or

GCQ-S (MacKenzie, 1983, 1990)—see Chapter 3. This easy to administer measure consists of 12 statements rated on seven-point Likert scales in terms of being relevant to a group session. Both patient and therapist formats exist. Eleven of the statements are collapsed to define three-dimensional scales: Engaged (describing group cohesion), Avoiding (indicating the reluctance of the group members to face their problems), and Conflict (indicating interpersonal friction). The 12th statement is a measure of general anxiety. The dimension scores for each session can be compared to patient or therapist means from a normative sample of 12 outpatient groups composed of non-psychotic patients.

In our study (Kanas and Barr, 1986), 34 consecutive sessions of a 45-minute triweekly inpatient integrative group for schizophrenia spectrum patients were evaluated by the two group leaders using the short form of the GCQ-S. All 22 patients who participated were male (13 white, 6 black, 3 Asian). During the three-month study period, sessions averaged six patients and two therapists. The average dimension scores are shown in the second column of Table 6.3.

Compared with the normative sample scores shown in column 6, there was no difference in the Avoiding dimension, but the integrative group scored significantly lower on a t-test in the Engaged (p < .02) and Conflict (p < .001) dimensions. The low-cohesion score was felt to be due to the rapid patient turnover characteristic of an inpatient versus outpatient setting, and the low amount of conflict likely reflected the group technique of encouraging safety and minimal expression of interpersonal anger in the integrative model. The mean anxiety score of 2.58 fell between the verbal descriptions of "somewhat" and "moderately" on the Likert scale for this item. A listing of topics discussed revealed that encouraging contact with others was most frequent during the sessions (discussed in 54 sessions), followed by expression of emotions (31 sessions) and reality testing (25 sessions). Advice-giving topics related to medication usage or discharge planning were last in frequency (18 sessions).

During a sabbatical in 1994, I conducted a process study of an inpatient schizophrenic group at a general hospital near London, UK (which

Table 6.3 GCQ-S mean dimension scores

Dimension	SFVA inpts. (Kanas and Barr, 1986)	British inpts. (Kanas unpub)	LPPI outpts. (Kanas, DiLella and Jones, 1984)	Short outpts. 1 LPPI, 2 SFVA (Kanas et al., 1989b)	Non-psychotic outpt. Norms (MacKenzie, 1983)
Engaged	12.79	16.80	14.46	14.86	14.61
Avoiding	9.74	5.70	11.46	7.66	10.33
Conflict	2.25	1.50	3.71	1.51	3.85

was introduced in Chapter 5). The integrative approach was taught to the staff, and I participated as a coleader in half of the sessions. The patients were from two open psychiatric units, where the average length of stay was about five weeks. The group met twice weekly for 45 minutes. Ten sessions were evaluated using the therapist form of the GCQ-S. Twelve male and eight female patients participated, and there were 10 black, 8 white, and 2 Asian patients. Each session averaged six patients and two therapists.

The GCQ-S dimension scores are shown in the third column of Table 6.3. Using t-tests, the British group scored significantly higher than the SFVA group in the Engaged dimension (p < .02) and significantly lower in the Avoiding dimension (p < .01). The Conflict score was lower but not significant. The mean anxiety score of 1.30 also was significantly lower (p < .001) than that in the SFVA group. Thus, the British group seemed to be more cohesive and less avoidant and tense than the American group. Factors contributing to these differences may have been the presence of females in the British group, who may have responded better to treatment and been more supportive than their male counterparts (Lazerson and Zilbach, 1993; Szymanski et al., 1995), and cultural differences between the two groups. In addition, fewer sessions were evaluated in the British study (10 vs. 34), which means that the patients were evaluated relatively early in their treatment (e.g., 75% of the British patients participated in only one to three sessions versus 36% in the SFVA sample, and 50% of the latter participated in more than eight sessions). MacKenzie believes that cohesion tends to be higher and avoidance lower in the earlier phases of a therapy group as patients bond around their common problems and haven't had time to develop the competitive conflicts characteristic of later sessions (MacKenzie, 1983, 1990; MacKenzie and Livesley, 1983). Consequently, it is possible that more of the British patients were in their group therapy "honeymoon period," and this may have accounted for their higher Engaged and lower Avoiding scores.

The topics discussed in the British group were reminiscent of the SFVA group. Of the 26 topics recorded, 11 dealt with ways to cope with hallucinations and delusions and 9 dealt with improving interpersonal relationships. Notably, these were congruent with the two main group goals of the integrative model, as discussed in Chapter 4.

Outpatient Studies

We also began using the integrative group model in the outpatient setting. The first study was conducted at an outpatient psychiatric clinic at the Langley Porter Psychiatric Institute (LPPI) of the University of California, San Francisco (UCSF) (Kanas, DiLella and Jones, 1984). Over the course of six months, 26 hourly sessions of weekly integrative group therapy were studied using the GCQ-S and a content analysis of discussion topics. The group was closed to new admissions after the fifth session, and throughout most of the study period, it was composed of six schizophrenia spectrum patients (four male and two female) and two male therapists, who were third-year UCSF psychiatric residents. I was the supervisor and observed all the sessions as a non-participant from outside the group circle. The overall attendance rate was 88%. In terms of the topics discussed, issues related to encouraging contact with others were most frequently discussed (in 32 sessions), followed by issues related to reality testing/coping with psychotic symptoms (19 sessions), expression of emotions (17 sessions), and advice-giving (10 sessions).

Using the therapist version of the GCQ-S, the overall scores on the three dimensions (fourth column of Table 6.3) did not differ significantly on t-tests from the means reported by MacKenzie (1983), shown in the last column of Table 6.3. Avoiding was higher but just missed being significant (p < .06). The anxiety score of 2.63 was between the "somewhat" and "moderately" descriptors.

We examined the session-by-session scores to look for evidence of group stages. There was a trend for the Avoiding scores to oscillate on the high side during the first 20 sessions and for the Engaged scores to increase and the Conflict scores to decrease over time. During the final seven sessions, Avoiding scores dropped and remained low, and a clear pattern of high Engaged scores and low Avoiding and Conflict scores resulted. In the MacKenzie system (MacKenzie, 1983, 1990; MacKenzie and Livesley, 1983), this pattern is consistent with either stage 1 of group development, where the group develops its identity and becomes more cohesive, or stage 3, where the members attempt to achieve an understanding of their problems through self-revelation and introspection. It is possible that this late pattern represented a delayed entry into, and subsequent fixation in, stage 1 of group development, as was suggested by the studies of Restek-Petrović et al. (2016) and Isbell, Thorne and Lawler (1992)—see Chapter 3. But another notion seems more in keeping with our data. Since Avoidance scores generally were high during the early part of the group, and since the integrative model calls for the group leaders to modulate intense affect expression (especially anger), it is possible that the group members avoided active consideration of their problems until they achieved some degree of comfort with one another. That is, they moved through attenuated stages 1 and 2 and coalesced into a clear pattern for stage 3. Indeed, during the last several sessions, the group members seemed more introspective, trusting of each other, and revealing in their discussions. This is consistent with clinical impressions, described in Chapter 4, that after four to six months, patients in integrative groups are able to discuss long-standing problems and maladaptive patterns of relating with others.

I became interested in trying the integrative group approach using a short-term format of 12 weekly, hourly outpatient group sessions. There were several reasons for this. Short-term groups are cost-effective and supported by managed care programs. They are more focused and clearer in their goals, and the therapists tend to be more directive (Klein, 1985), notions that seemed congruent with the integrative model. Since psychotic conditions tend to be long-term, patients could be treated by a series of repeated short-term group experiences. This would satisfy yearly session limitations of some managed care providers, give psychotic patients non-group intervals to test out what they have learned, and provide them with a sense of both beginning and ending a planned treatment course, rare for these individuals.

With these notions in mind, the first short-term group study was conducted at an outpatient clinic at the LPPI (Kanas, Stewart and Haney, 1988). I coled the group with a third-year UCSF psychiatric resident. The group met hourly for 12 consecutive weekly sessions. There were two major group goals: helping the schizophrenia spectrum patients improve their relationships and helping them learn ways of testing reality and coping with their symptoms (i.e., hallucinations, delusions, and loose associations). Seven patients started but two dropped out by the third session (one was hospitalized to stabilize his board and care situation). Five patients completed the group (three male, four white, one black), and the attendance rate was 80%. The patients completed several outcome measures at the beginning and end of the 12-week trial, including the discharge questionnaire used in an earlier study (Kanas and Barr, 1982)—see Figure 6.1. A nurse-observer recorded the discussion topics.

There were no significant pre-post group differences on the 90-item Symptom Checklist (SCL-90) or the Brief Psychiatric Rating Scale. However, a t-test revealed a significant improvement ($p < .05$) on the Social Avoidance and Distress scale (SAD). This suggested that the patients became more comfortable relating with others as a result of their group experience. The fact that they were being medicated also could be a factor.

On the discharge questionnaire, all members rated the group as "very" or "somewhat" helpful. The rank order of therapeutic factors is shown in Table 6.4. Note that the point distribution is less varied than for the inpatient study (compare with Table 6.1). In fact, there were no differences greater than one point among adjacent ranked items, so if only one person had altered his or her score, the ranking would have been changed. Thus, one must discuss the results with caution. Also, the presence of tied rankings makes statistical comparisons difficult. Nevertheless, using three standard measures of correlation (Pearson's r, Spearman's rho, and Kendall's tau), the two rankings in Table 6.4 and Table 6.1 correlate significantly at $p < .001$ (Vasavada, 2016). This is to be expected, since the therapy groups derive from the same clinical model. One observation is that the five highest ranked statements in this study were among the six highest ranking statements in the inpatient study. Thus, for these two short-term groups, relating better with others, testing reality, and coping

Table 6.4 Ranking of therapeutic factors in a short-term outpatient group
(Kanas et al., 1988)

Therapeutic factor statement	Points	Rank
The group helped me become less suspicious of others.	9	1
The group taught me how to relate better with people.	8	2
The group helped me decide the difference between reality and my imagination.	8	2
The group showed me that I am not the only one with problems.	7	4
The group showed me that I can help other people.	7	4
The group helped me feel hopeful about my future.	6	6
The group allowed me a place to express my emotions.	5	7
The group helped me cope better with my voices and/or visions.	4	8
The group gave me insight into the causes of my problems.	4	8
The group gave me useful advice about the nature of my illness.	4	8
The group gave me useful advice about medications.	4	8
The group helped me learn to control some of my emotions.	3	12
The group gave me useful advice about jobs, finances, or places to stay.	3	12

with psychotic experiences were rated higher than gaining insight or receiving advice about their illness or medications.

This paralleled the content analysis of discussion topics, where issues relating to relationships (discussed 21 times) and reality testing/coping with psychotic symptoms (15 times) were considered more often than issues related to advice-giving (12 times), the group itself (12 times), or the expression of emotions (11 times).

Four months after completing this group, the patients were contacted by phone and asked several structured questions about their ability to relate with others and cope with psychotic symptoms. Four of the five patients reported gains in their ability to interact with others, and two believed that they were coping better with psychotic symptoms. None of the patients had been hospitalized or received significant changes in their clinical care. Three felt that the group had been just right in length, and two said it was too short.

This study was followed by a controlled study involving two time-limited, 12-session hourly groups in an outpatient clinic at the SFVA (Kanas et al., 1989a). Fourteen patients began the groups and 12 finished: all had schizophrenia spectrum diagnoses, 11 were males, 8 were white, and 4 were black. The two groups were coled by me and a third-year UCSF psychiatric resident. The patient attendance rate was 89%, and discussion topics were recorded throughout the sessions. An additional nine patients were assigned to a waiting list control condition; they did not differ demographically from the group patients. All patients were given the SCL-90 and the SAD at the beginning and end of the four-month group or control condition. All of the patients were contacted after four months of a no-group therapy follow-up period and were asked a series of questions similar to those used in our previous LPPI outpatient study (Kanas, Stewart and Haney, 1988).

On the SCL-90, the scores for the group patients dropped on all nine symptom dimensions, and two of these decreases (anxiety and somatization) were significant using an analysis of variance when compared with the waiting list control patients. The group patient SAD scores also dropped, but this failed to reach significance. Group discussion topics dealing with relationships were brought up most frequently (25 times in the two groups), followed by reality testing/coping with psychotic symptoms (18 times), topics pertaining to the group itself (17 times), the expression of emotions (seven times), and advice-giving (six times).

During the four-month follow-up interviews, the group patients rated their previous group experiences as "very" or "somewhat" helpful. Nine thought that the group was about right in duration, and three said it was too short. Six stated that they would like to participate in a similar group in the future. In response to questions assessing their clinical status in 10 dimensions during the four months of no-group activity, there were no significant interval differences recorded using the Fisher exact test between the group and control patients in the following eight areas: general psychological problems, antipsychotic medication dose, hospitalization status, outpatient therapy time, living arrangements, job or disability status, legal status, or physical condition. However, there were significant differences in two areas, as shown in Table 6.5.

Compared with the waiting list control patients, the group patients experienced significant increases in relating better with other people and coping with psychotic symptoms. This is notable because these are the two areas that the therapists were told to focus on in the group, and they matched the topics most commonly discussed. This suggests that a focused 12-session group therapy experience with clear goals can impact on schizophrenia spectrum patients for at least four months after the group

Table 6.5 Significant follow-up dimension scores: group versus control patients (Kanas et al., 1989a)

Dimension	Short-term group pts. (%)	Waiting list control pts. (%)	p-value
Relating better with other people	88	11	.01
Coping better with psychotic symptoms	63	0	.03

ends in the areas of improved relationships and coping with psychotic symptoms.

The three 12-session groups mentioned above (one LPPI and two SFVA) all were evaluated using the therapist version of the GCQ-S (Kanas et al., 1989b). The intra-class correlation coefficient revealed that the therapist interrater reliabilities across the groups were good, and patients did not differ significantly in terms of sex, race, and diagnoses. The three dimensional scores did not differ among the three groups, with the exception of one of the SFVA groups that scored significantly higher than the other two on the Engaged dimension. This unusually cohesive group had no dropouts and a much higher attendance rate than the other two (99%). But despite this one high score, the mean Engaged score for the three short-term outpatient groups was not different from MacKenzie's outpatient normative sample, as is shown in columns 5 and 6 of Table 6.3. However, the short-term mean scores were significantly lower than the normative sample for the Avoiding (p < .001) and Conflict (p < .001) dimensions. Again, this suggests that the groups were safe and that strong emotions, especially those leading to conflict, were moderated.

Similar to the long-term outpatient group described earlier (Kanas, DiLella and Jones, 1984), there was a tendency for the Engaged scores to increase and the Avoiding and Conflict scores to decrease as time went on. However, there was no clear pattern of high Engaged and low Avoiding and Conflict across several sequential sessions as there was in the earlier long-term group.

The three groups averaged five patients per session, the average dropout rate was 19%, and the overall attendance rate was 86%; all respectable values for a therapy group.

After two years, all the SFVA-eligible patients in these three groups were invited to participate in another 12-session "repeaters group" at the SFVA (Kanas and Smith, 1990). Of the 12 eligible patients contacted, seven (58%) agreed to participate. One dropped out after the third session, but the remaining six (all schizophrenia spectrum, one white woman, three white men, two black men) completed the group. As with all of the outpatient time-limited groups, the patients met weekly for one hour, and the group was closed to new admissions once it began. Each session averaged 5.6 patients and two therapists, and the attendance rate was 89%. At the end of the 12 sessions, five patients rated the group as "very" helpful, and 1 said it was "somewhat" helpful (Kanas, 1991).

The two therapists (me and an SFVA psychology intern) felt that the patients bonded quickly and dealt with interpersonal issues and symptom-coping strategies more efficiently than was the case in the earlier groups. That is, they seemed to pick up where they left off in their earlier group experience. They were able to consider more sophisticated problem areas, such as examining the role of long-standing maladaptive patterns of interpersonal behavior throughout their lives in fostering suspicions and fear of relationships. Again, this is consistent with our clinical notions that psychotic patients in integrative outpatient group therapy are able to deal with topics related to long-standing problems and maladaptive patterns of relating with others after four and six months.

Because all 12 sessions of the repeaters group were videotaped, a trained rater scored them using the HIM-G (Kanas and Smith, 1990). Since session 8 had no sound, recordings could only be made of the other 11 sessions. The fourth column of Table 6.2 shows the mean percentile scores of these sessions for the content and work styles. Again, the uniqueness of the integrative model was shown only in the Confrontive work style, with a percentile score of 98. Similar to the two inpatient studies referred to in Table 6.2 (Kanas, Barr and Dossick, 1985; Kanas and Smith, 1990), the Topic/Confrontive matrix cell also was unique at the 99th+ percentile. According to the Spearman Rank-Order Correlation, the ranking of the 16 matrix cells correlated significantly with the inpatient groups reported in both the 1985 study (p < .001) and the 1990 report (p < .001). Also, similar to the inpatient groups, patients in the repeaters 12-session outpatient group failed to react to the therapists only 5%–10% of the time, and total group resistance was low at 1%–5% of overall group activity. The therapists were active, accounting for 26% of the group time. As in the other groups, they were especially active in the Confrontive area, which had the highest Th/M category ratio of 1.36. Thus, the same factors making the integrative model unique in the inpatient setting appeared to apply in the short-term outpatient setting as well.

Recently, I evaluated the characteristics of a long-term outpatient integrative group using the questionnaire shown in Figure 6.1, which is similar to that used in the VA short-term inpatient group (Kanas and Barr, 1982—see Table 6.1) and the LPPI short-term outpatient group (Kanas, Stewart and Haney, 1988—see Table 6.4), reported above. This group was conducted in a mental health outpatient clinic and met weekly for 45-minute sessions. I led the group, along with several rotating nurse practitioner and psychology intern students who functioned as coleaders. The integrative treatment model was very similar to that used in the earlier studies, except that there were additional psychoeducational and CBT presentations incorporated into appropriate discussions that used a white board to describe the A–B–C cognitive model and the vulnerability-stress model (see Chapter 2) and the "U" curve external stimulation-symptom relationship (see Vignette 4.9, Chapter 4). In fact, these changes prompted my clinical evaluation, since I was curious to see if the patients would perceive the group environment differently as a result of these additions to the model.

The evaluation period was from January to December 2019. A total of 47 sessions were included that involved 11 patients with schizophrenia spectrum diagnoses. Five of the patients had started the group the year before and three of these continued throughout all of 2019. The other six patients were added during the course of the year. Overall, four of the patients terminated treatment during the year, two when the time of the group had to change and they couldn't attend the new time, and two because they moved out of the state. Of those patients who were active during the evaluation period (one patient missed several sessions due to an excused medical and housing problem, but later returned), the mean attendance rate was 79.5%, and the mean number of patients per session was 5.0. No one was hospitalized for psychiatric reasons during that calendar year.

I was interested in looking at the group experience of the patients who attended for a long period of time. Seven patients attended 20 or more sessions of the group, and the mean total number of sessions attended was 30.6. All seven completed the discharge questionnaire (Figure 6.1) when they left the group or at the end of December 2019. All respondents rated the group as being "very helpful."

The results of the therapeutic factor section of the discharge questionnaire are shown in Table 6.6. Note that like the short-term outpatient ranking shown in Table 6.4, the distribution of points for the first 10 ranked statements clustered closely together, with adjacent items not differing by more than one point; so again, one must be cautious in discussing

Table 6.6 Ranking of therapeutic factors in a long-term outpatient group

Therapeutic factor statement	Points	Ranking
The group gave me useful advice about the nature of my illness.	13	1
The group showed me that I am not the only one with problems.	13	1
The group allowed me a place to express my emotions.	12	3
The group taught me how to relate better with people.	12	3
The group showed me that I can help other people.	12	3
The group helped me feel hopeful about my future.	12	3
The group helped me decide the difference between reality and my imagination.	11	7
The group gave me insight into the causes of my problems.	10	8
The group helped me learn to control some of my emotions.	10	8
The group helped me cope better with my voices and/or visions.	9.5	10
The group gave me useful advice about medications.	7	11
The group helped me become less suspicious of others.	6	12
The group me useful advice about jobs, finances, or places to stay.	5	13

the rankings. Using three standard measures of correlation (Pearson's r, Spearman's rho, and Kendall's tau), the two rankings in Table 6.6 and Table 6.4 correlated significantly at p < .001 (Vasavada, 2016). Similarly, the two rankings in Table 6.6 and Table 6.1 also correlated significantly at p < .001. Five of the top seven items in the long-term group appeared in the top six rankings in the short-term inpatient group (Table 6.1) and in the top seven rankings of the short-term outpatient group (Table 6.4). Also note that the item related to receiving useful advice about jobs, finances, or places to stay was rated last in all three studies.

Despite the general similarity among the three groups, the long-term group showed two interesting differences. First, the top-rated therapeutic factors in the long-term group clustered more toward relating better with others and expressing emotions than coping with symptoms such as hallucinations and delusions, which were relatively low. This supports the notion presented in Chapter 4 (see Tables 4.6 and 4.7) that long-term integrative psychosis groups start to look more like non-psychotic groups as the patients learn to trust each other and move beyond discussions of coping with hallucinations and delusions in favor of more emotional and interpersonal issues. Second, receiving useful advice about the nature of their illness shot up to number 1 in the long-term group from its lower rankings (numbers 8 and 10) in the two short-term groups. I believe that this is less a factor of group duration than the fact that more psychoeducational and CBT presentations were incorporated into the treatment method over the past few years (e.g., A–B–C cognitive model, vulnerability-stress model, "U" curve external stimulation-symptom relationship). These changes likely were appreciated by the patients in helping them increase their understanding of their psychotic disease.

Lessons Learned

The body of research on the outcome and process of the integrative group therapy model has consisted of a number of small studies conducted over a long period of time. Although some of these studies were uncontrolled, most had either a no-group control condition or compared results with a published normative sample of therapy groups not using the integrative method. Significant findings resulted that supported the safety and value of the integrative model. Furthermore, many findings were replicated in separate studies done years apart and in different settings, again lending credence to this approach.

What can we conclude from these studies? In terms of *outcome*, psychotic inpatients have rated the integrative group experience as being helpful at the time of discharge, especially younger and non-paranoid patients. Ward staff also have noted improvements in these patients. In the outpatient setting, the integrative model has been well-received in both long-term and short-term formats. Attendance rates typically are in the

80%–90% range, and drop-out rates are under 20%. In studies of three 12-session, time-limited, outpatient integrative groups, some psychotic patients experienced symptom reduction, a lowering of social anxiety, and improvement in their relationships with others. In one study, improvements in social relationships and symptom coping strategies were found to exist four months after the group ended when compared to a waiting list control sample of similar patients.

The majority of outpatients who completed a short-term, 12-session integrative group trial choose to participate in a similar group within two years. For those who desired additional therapy, regularly attending sequential short-term repeaters groups or a long-term closed group presents chronic psychotic patients with viable treatment options. For patients who felt that one course of treatment was enough, the experience of successfully terminating a therapeutic activity may have served to increase their confidence and prevent unnecessary treatment dependency, although this was not formally evaluated.

In studies of the integrative group *process* in both inpatient and outpatient settings, the members were found to engage in high quality work, show low levels of avoidance and conflict, and confront significant aspects of their problems with minimal resistance and anxiety. In one study at a hospital in England, an inpatient group based on my model scored significantly higher than an inpatient group in America on a measure of cohesion and significantly lower on measures of avoidance and anxiety, possibly reflecting gender and cultural differences in the two samples. Outpatient integrative groups show a pattern of increased cohesion and decreased avoidance and conflict as time goes on. There was no evidence of the kind of conflict observed in the second stage of group development that is found in many therapy groups with non-psychotic patients. The therapists were active and successful in shaping the parameters of the group that were most congruent with the group goals.

Generally, psychotic patients valued the integrative groups more as a place to learn strategies of interacting with others, of testing reality and coping with psychotic symptoms, and of expressing emotions than as a place to develop insight and to receive advice concerning their illness, medications, or economic situation. However, in a long-term group using this model, valued therapeutic factors clustered a bit more toward relating better with others and expressing emotions than coping with symptoms such as hallucinations and delusions. This suggests that these patients already had learned much about coping strategies and now were prepared to discuss and gain insight into long-standing problems and maladaptive patterns of relating with others, which clinically I have found to occur after four to six months. They also appreciated the addition of new psychoeducational and CBT elements, which gave them more information about their illness.

References

Hill, W.F. (1961) *Hill Interaction Matrix (HIM) Scoring Manual.* Los Angeles: Youth Studies Center, University of Southern California.

Hill, W.F. (1965) *Hill Interaction Matrix (HIM) Monograph.* Los Angeles: Youth Studies Center, University of Southern California.

Isbell, S.E., Thorne, A. and Lawler, M.H. (1992) An exploratory study of video-tapes of long-term group psychotherapy of outpatients with major and chronic mental illness. *Group,* 16, 101–111.

Kanas, N. (1991) Group therapy with schizophrenic patients: A short-term, homogeneous approach. *International Journal of Group Psychotherapy,* 41, 33–48.

Kanas, N. and Barr, M.A. (1982) Short-term homogeneous group therapy for schizophrenic inpatients: A questionnaire evaluation. *Group,* 6(4), 32–38.

Kanas, N. and Barr, M.A. (1983) Homogeneous group therapy for acutely psychotic schizophrenic inpatients. *Hospital and Community Psychiatry,* 34(3), 257–259.

Kanas, N. and Barr, M.A. (1986) Process and content in a short-term inpatient schizophrenic group. *Small Group Behavior,* 17, 355–363.

Kanas, N., Barr, M.A. and Dossick, S. (1985) The homogeneous schizophrenic inpatient group: An evaluation using the Hill Interaction Matrix. *Small Group Behavior,* 16, 397–409.

Kanas, N. and Smith, A.J. (1990) Schizophrenic group process: A comparison and replication using the HIM-G. *Group,* 14(4), 246–252.

Kanas, N., Deri, J., Ketter, T. and Fein, G. (1989a) Short-term outpatient therapy groups for schizophrenics. *International Journal of Group Psychotherapy,* 39, 517–522.

Kanas, N., DiLella, V.J. and Jones, J. (1984) Process and content in an outpatient schizophrenic group. *Group,* 8(2), 13–20.

Kanas, N., Stewart, P., Deri, J., Ketter, T. and Haney, K. (1989b) Group process in short-term outpatient therapy groups for schizophrenics. *Group,* 13(2), 67–73.

Kanas, N., Stewart, P. and Haney, K. (1988) Content and outcome in a short-term therapy group for schizophrenic outpatients. *Hospital and Community Psychiatry,* 39(4), 437–439.

Klein, R.H. (1985) Some principles of short-term group psychotherapy. *International Journal of Group Psychotherapy,* 35, 309–330.

Lazerson, J.S. and Zilbach, J.J. (1993) Gender issues in group psychotherapy. In: H.I. Kaplan and B.J. Sadock (Eds.), *Comprehensive Group Psychotherapy,* 3rd ed. Baltimore, MD: Williams & Wilkins, pp. 682–693.

MacKenzie, K.R. (1983) The clinical application of a group climate measure. In: R.R. Dies and K.R. Makenzie (Eds.), *Advances in Group Psychotherapy: Integrating Research and Practice.* New York: International Universities Press, pp. 159–170.

MacKenzie, K.R. (1990) *Introduction to Time-Limited Group Psychotherapy.* Washington, D.C.: American Psychiatric Press.

MacKenzie, K.R. and Livesley, W.J. (1983) A developmental model for brief group therapy. In: R.R. Dies and K.R. Makenzie (Eds.), *Advances in Group Psychotherapy: Integrating Research and Practice.* New York: International Universities Press, pp. 101–116.

Restek-Petrović, B., Gregurek, R., Petrović, R., Orešković-Krezler, N., Mihanović, M. and Ivezić, E. (2016) Characteristics of the group process in long-term psychodynamic group psychotherapy for patients with psychosis. *International Journal of Group Psychotherapy*, 66, 132–143.

Szymanski, S., Lieberman, J.A., Alvir, J.M., ... Cooper, T. (1995) Gender differences in onset of illness, treatment response, course, and biological indexes in first-episode schizophrenic patients. *American Journal of Psychiatry*, 152, 698–703.

Vasavada, N. (2016) https://astatsa.com/CorrelationTest/.

Yalom, I.D. (1975) *The Theory and Practice of Group Psychotherapy*, 2nd ed. New York: Basic Books.

7 Integrative Groups for Non-Psychotic Bipolar Patients

Introduction

In the preceding chapters, the focus has been on patients with psychotic symptoms, mostly those with schizophrenia spectrum disorders (e.g., schizophrenia, schizoaffective disorder, delusional disorder), but also people suffering from bipolar disorder and unspecified conditions, where psychosis continues to plague them. In this chapter, I will discuss therapy groups based on the integrative model for the majority of bipolar patients who, when not acutely ill, do not have continuing psychosis. In these so-called euthymic individuals, extremes of mania and depression are not present, although many have difficulty modulating their emotional state and worry about having future acute breakdowns.

Nature of Bipolar Disorder

Bipolar disorder (previously called manic-depressive disease) is an episodic condition characterized by disturbances in mood. Two forms are recognized in the DSM-5: bipolar I and bipolar II (American Psychiatric Association, 2013). The essential feature of bipolar I disorder is a history of at least one manic episode. Often, patients with this condition have had periods of depression as well. In bipolar II disorder, the clinical course is characterized by at least one major depressive episode and at least one period of hypomania. Both forms are characterized by recurrent episodes, with a strong genetic predisposition affecting first-degree biological relatives at a rate higher than normally expected (American Psychiatric Association, 2013).

In their survey taken from 9,282 respondents in the United States, Merikangas and her colleagues (2007) found the lifetime prevalences to be 1.0% for bipolar I disorder, 1.1% for bipolar II disorder, and 2.4% for sub-threshold bipolar disorder (which they defined as recurrent hypomania without a major depressive episode or with fewer symptoms than required for full-blown threshold hypomania). Prevalences were higher for women for BP-I and BP-II and higher for men for sub-threshold bipolar disorder. Using DSM-IV criteria, the authors found that comorbidity with other lifetime Axis I disorders (especially anxiety disorders) is the norm for both threshold (95.8%–97.7%) and sub-threshold (88.4%) bipolar disorders.

The major treatment for bipolar disorder is pharmacotherapy, usually involving lithium and other mood stabilizers, but sometime necessitating antipsychotic medications (Kaplan and Sadock, 1989). Unfortunately, about one-third of patients with mood disorders do not adhere fully to their prescribed medication regimen (Rahmani et al., 2016; Scott and Pope, 2002). In many cases, this is because they feel better once the acute phase of their illness subsides, and they see no need to continue with the prescribed pharmacotherapy. Unfortunately, sub-optimal adherence to medication is associated with significant increases in rehospitalizations (Rahmani et al., 2016; Scott and Pope, 2002) and sometimes even suicide. Bieling, McCabe and Antony (2009) cite a report stating that 15%–46% of bipolar patients do not comply with their pharmacological regimen, and they believe that this issue must be addressed directly in treatment.

Sajatovic, Davies and Hrouda (2004) did a literature review involving bipolar patients that measured adherence to either mood-stabilizing medications or psychotherapy. Seven of the 11 controlled studies that met their criteria for inclusion found that the chosen psychosocial intervention improved treatment adherence among bipolar patients. Interventions that were effective included interpersonal group therapy, cognitive-behavior therapy (CBT), group sessions for partners of patients with bipolar disorder, and patient and family psychoeducation. Important treatment issues that helped with pharmacotherapy adherence, included a good understanding of medications and their risks and benefits and education involving illness awareness and self-management. Most effective treatments featured an interactional component between patients and their care providers or therapists.

Traditionally, patients with bipolar disorder have been viewed as difficult to treat in group therapy, especially when in a manic phase (Yalom, 1975). During these times, they may be intrusive, hyperactive, irritable, impatient, and disruptive. Their thoughts are speeded up and tangential, and they often have grandiose delusions. The stimulation of being in a room with other people makes their symptoms worse, and most treatment approaches put manic patients in a low-stimulation environment, such as in a quiet room, where stimulation is kept to a minimum. For these reasons, group therapy is contraindicated for acutely manic patients.

Bipolar patients are more manageable in a therapy group when they are in a mildly depressed or euthymic state, which is defined as "a stable mental state or mood in those affected with bipolar disorder that is neither manic nor depressive" (Merriam-Webster Medical Dictionary, 2019). Nevertheless, they still represent therapeutic challenges. They tend to deny their problems and often exhibit poor interpersonal skills. In addition, the presence of genetic and constitutional factors and the success of lithium and other mood-stabilizing medications lead many clinicians (and the patient themselves) to conceptualize bipolar disorder as a biological disease and psychopharmacological treatment as the only treatment approach. Psychotherapy often is considered unimportant for these patients. But as we shall see, not all bipolar patients achieve optimal stability with medications alone, and there is evidence to support the notion that bipolar patients may benefit from group therapy, especially if it is used in conjunction with mood-stabilizing medications. Many approaches address psychodynamic and interpersonal issues that are problematic for these patients, but psychoeducation and cognitive-behavioral approaches also have been used. These now will be reviewed, with particular reference to group therapy. As in the earlier chapters of this book dealing with groups for psychotic patients, the following will be divided into non-didactic and didactic approaches.

Non-Didactic Approaches: Psychoanalytic/Psychodynamic and Interpersonal Issues

Theoretical Background

In an intensive psychoanalytic study of 12 manic-depressive (bipolar) patients, anxiety and conflict were seen as occurring during a later stage of oral development (Cohen et al., 1954; Gibson, Cohen and Cohen, 1959). This is the period when relating to others as individuals separate from one's self is forming. Failure to normally progress through this period can result in a dependent state, where the individual exhibits a poor ability to integrate concepts of the good and bad mother into a single person and exhibits a poor self-concept. Their strong dependence on others and their increased separation anxiety make these patients cautious in their expression of anger and superficial in their relationships. Many deny these painful feelings and react with compensatory overconfidence and grandiose ideas.

In addition, the families of people with bipolar disorder often differ demographically from others in their surroundings (e.g., racially, economically). This results in upwardly mobile pressures on the children and excessive adherence to conventional standards. In some cases, the mother was the more driving and ambitious parent, whereas the father was less effectual and blamed by the mother for the family's problems. Consequently, the developing child was encouraged to deny feelings, engage in envious and competitive relationships, and orient values in terms of social conventions.

These pressures continue into adulthood, resulting in a situation where dependency needs and family insecurities are denied, and a compensatory aggressiveness and desire to succeed in a conventional manner become overt, especially when dependency needs are activated. Depressive episodes are seen as intensifications of the emptiness felt internally, and manic episodes are seen as a denial and defense against this painful emotional state (Kanas, 1993).

These concepts were tested in a study involving 39 manic-depressive patients and 17 schizophrenic patients (Gibson, 1958; Gibson, Cohen and Cohen, 1959). The bipolar patients scored significantly higher on scales measuring envy, conventionality, and relationships to the community, and their specific scores on envy, competitiveness, and pressure to conform socially were particularly high. In addition, the bipolar patients were more likely to come from families who were trying to rise socioeconomically and who used their children to further this familial goal, rather than treating them as individuals in their own right. Thus, there is some empirical support for the classical psychoanalytical formulation characterizing these individuals, and this gives credence to the notion that dynamically oriented therapeutic approaches may be of value for bipolar patients.

Important interpersonal issues also have been evaluated in case studies involving bipolar patients. Janowsky, Leff and Epstein (1970) studied 15 acutely manic inpatients and isolated five characteristics that served their need to control other people. These were manipulation of others' self-esteem to gain interpersonal leverage; ability to recognize vulnerability and internal conflicts, which placed others on the defensive; denial and projection of responsibility, which resulted in other people feeling guilty for the manic patient's actions; frequent testing of limits by making incrementally larger requests of others; and alienation of family and friends through these and other interpersonal maneuvers. The authors noted that this last characteristic affected the therapeutic relationship, resulting in countertransferential nihilism, over-prescribing of medications, and a desire by the therapist to see the patient shift to a more manageable depressive state.

Some of these interpersonal ideas were supported in a study involving 29 inpatients suffering from a number of psychotic disorders (Janowsky, El-Yousef and Davis, 1974). The bipolar subjects scored significantly higher than the others on measures evaluating limit-testing, projection of responsibility, sensitivity to others' vulnerabilities, splitting of staff, flattering behavior, and ability to provoke anger. Interestingly, the scores diminished as the patients were treated and became more euthymic.

O'Connell and colleagues (1985) studied psychosocial factors in 60 bipolar patients who were treated with lithium for one year. Outcome measures scored for number of affective episodes, social adjustment, and global assessment. The factor found to correlate most highly with positive outcome was social support, which the authors viewed as the resources, relationships, and structures available to the patients to serve as positive buffers to negative life experiences.

Non-Didactic Group Therapy: Clinical Implications

Many of the above psychodynamic and interpersonal issues have been described in therapy groups involving bipolar patients. Ablon et al. (1975) reported that many of their group patients had poor contact with their fathers as children due to disinterest, frequent business separations, or even death. As adults, the men in their study tended to identify with their weak and absent fathers and ended up marrying dominant women. In contrast, the bipolar women identified with their dominant mothers and married men who were passive or absent like their fathers. Interestingly, the men more often had intact marriages than the women.

Volkmar et al. (1981) noted that bipolar patients in group therapy described problems with dependency, anger, and impulsivity. They tended to use denial as a typical defense mechanism. Since most of their patients were euthymic, these characteristics were viewed as personality traits rather than being part of an extreme mood swing. Interpersonally, the group members were conventional and sociable externally, which the authors believed served to defend against true intimacy.

Pollack (1990) reported on a psychotherapy group for bipolar inpatients that met weekly for 50-minute sessions. The group format was interpersonally oriented but structured to accommodate the rapid patient turnover of the unit. The author concluded that the patients were able to interact effectively in the group, discuss factors related to the nature of their illness, consider ways of coping with it, and consider strategies of improving their interpersonal relationships.

Finally, Cerbone et al. (1992) reported that their bipolar group patients exhibited decline in work and interpersonal performance, even when they were euthymic. This was felt to result from developmental disruptions in identity and capacity for intimacy that normally would occur during late adolescence or early adulthood, which was a time that many of their patients began to exhibit symptoms of their disorder.

Non-Didactic Group Therapy: Research Findings

Several research studies have supported the value of non-didactic therapy groups for bipolar patients when used in conjunction with mood-stabilizing medications. One such study examined the effect of couples' group therapy on a subgroup of 65 bipolar patients who were admitted to a National Institute of Mental Health (NIMH) research ward for treatment of acute mania (Ablon et al., 1975; Davenport et al., 1977). After being stabilized, these patients were followed for two to ten years after discharge for medication management. Twelve married patients received weekly couples' group therapy that was nondirective and supportive. They were compared with 11 similar patients who received medication management only at NIMH, and another 42 patients who were referred back to their home communities for management of their mood-stabilizing medications. During the follow-up period, the couples' group patients did better than the others in terms of number of readmissions, marital failures, global functioning, and family interactions.

In another study (Shakir et al., 1979; Volkmar et al., 1981), 20 outpatients at a Department of Veterans Affairs (VA) clinic who had bipolar disorder were followed in a psychotherapy group that met weekly for 75 minutes. The format used an interactional, interpersonal, here-and-now approach based on Yalom (1975) that focused on the expression of affect, reality issues, current problems related to their illness, and improving interpersonal relationships. Patients were followed for up to four years and averaged 47 sessions of group therapy. Comparing the two-year period after beginning the group with the two years prior to entry, the number of weeks of hospitalization dropped from 16.8 to 3.6 per year, and the number of patients in continuous full-time employment increased from 6 to 16.

Kripke and Robinson (1985) reported on their over ten-year experience with a bipolar psychotherapy group that met at a VA outpatient clinic. A total of 17 patients were involved with the group. The original goal was to provide a forum to supervise lithium management, but gradually, the patients bonded together and began meeting biweekly for 1½-hour sessions. Initially, the two therapists encouraged self-revelation and psychodynamic analysis of group interactions, but later they found that problem-solving discussions of current difficulties were more useful. Medication and blood-level reviews were made at the beginning of the sessions. An interesting feature of the program was an annual potluck dinner involving the patients and their families, during which the therapists gave a presentation on the use of lithium, and family members were encouraged to share their feelings about having a bipolar family member. At the end of the study period, 8 of the original 14 group members still were involved. The authors reported that the rate of hospitalizations of patients decreased, and the socioeconomic function of five group members improved since entering the group.

Wulsin, Bachop and Hoffman (1988) conducted a psychotherapy group for bipolar patients that meet for 4½ years in a community mental health setting. The focus of the weekly group was to encourage the patients to discuss the effects of their illness on their relationships with others, with particular reference to issues they faced in dealing with the management of their disease. The patients had their blood lithium levels monitored by clinicians who were not involved with the group. The authors concluded that the 22 patients who participated in the group benefited from the experience and related to one another in a cohesive manner, despite a relatively high dropout rate of 55%.

Cerbone et al. (1992) conducted an outpatient study of 43 bipolar patients on lithium who were treated in a weekly therapy group that met for 75-minute sessions. The group used educational, supportive, and counseling techniques to help the members confront denial, understand their illness, and improve their relationships with others. Compared to the year prior to entering the group, the patients experienced significant improvement in ratings of severity and duration of affective episodes, school and work productivity, interpersonal functioning, and mean number and days of hospitalization during the year following their enrollment. There were no significant changes in medication usage.

Hallensleben (1994) reported on her ten years' experience leading a bipolar group. The therapeutic approach was eclectic, ranging from supportive and structuring interventions with new patients to insight-stimulating interventions with older group members. She concluded that the patients became more self-supporting and autonomous as a result of their group experience, and she found that their rehospitalization rate was reduced. In two separate evaluations made in 1988 and 1991, over 80% of the respondents indicated that they had benefitted from their group experience.

Didactic Approaches: Psychoeducational and Cognitive-Behavioral Issues

Theoretical Background

Didactic approaches to bipolar disorder emphasize the genetic/constitutional and phenomenological aspects of the disease rather than its psychodynamic or interpersonal manifestations. The focus is on educating these patients about the nature and course of the disorder (discussed previously in this chapter), alerting them to prodromal symptoms of an impending acute episode, helping them contain and modify behaviors associated with the signs and symptoms of the disease, supporting cognitive shifts away from the despair of depression and the exuberance of mania, and teaching bipolar patients the importance of complying with prescribed medications (particularly lithium and other mood stabilizers).

Bieling, McCabe and Antony (2009) view the mood swings in bipolar disorder as two opposing sides of the same coin. In mania, a person sees him- or herself, the world, and the future in unrealistically glowing and positive terms. In depression, these characteristics are their exact opposite: unrealistically pessimistic and negative. The authors feel that such unrealistic thoughts and beliefs can be subjected to cognitive techniques involving reality testing and consideration of multiple perspectives. Furthermore, since external stressors play an important role in triggering both depression and mania, reducing the frequency and intensity of such stressors is also an important goal of treatment. Finally, since poor medication compliance is a problem in bipolar patients psychoeducational techniques aimed at understanding the nature of their illness, and the need for pharmacological intervention are critical.

Didactic Group Therapy: Clinical Implications

In an early report on group CBT, Palmer, Williams and Adams (1995) describe a manualized, structured method of treating medicated bipolar patients in groups comprised 17 weekly, 90-minute sessions. Topics dealt with identifying and correcting negative thoughts and cognitive distortions related to depression as well as hyper-positive thoughts and flare-ups related to manic episodes. Circadian rhythm disorganization also was considered. Techniques included lectures, in-group exercises, and discussions of homework assignments. Participants were evaluated on several self-report measures of symptomatology, social adjustment, and mood, and their hospitalization and consultation histories were recorded in the 12 months prior to and after treatment. Although six bipolar patients began the program, only four completed it, so it was difficult to generalize about treatment effectiveness. However, all showed improvement on some of the symptomatology and social adjustment subscales, suggesting that this approach was useful for bipolar patients and that further controlled studies were warranted.

Bieling, McCabe and Antony (2009) have proposed a manualized group treatment approach for bipolar patients that consider the psychoeducational, cognitive, behavioral, and stress-responsive needs of bipolar patients. Their approach consists of 17 weekly sessions, each of which meets for two hours, followed by three monthly "booster" sessions. The first two sessions involve educational presentations about the illness and the use of medications, followed by questions and discussions. Families are invited to these sessions. The next four sessions consider behavioral strategies for dealing with depression and mania and, like subsequent sessions, include exercises and homework assignments. Prodromal symptoms and behavioral changes are identified, such as disruption of sleep and decreased or increased energy, and patients are taught good sleep hygiene, strategies to deal with stimulation, and non-pharmaceutical relaxation techniques, such as yoga and exercise. The next six sessions deal with cognitive issues, such as recognizing the kinds of thoughts that typically accompany mood states and employing alternative ways of thinking to counter negativity or hyper-positivity. Thought records are made to enhance the group discussions. Specific problem-solving techniques and coping strategies are considered in the next two sessions. Action plans are introduced in response to the thought records. The final three sessions deal with the identification of underlying cognitive beliefs and schemas that contribute to the illness as well as to a sense of defectiveness and shame perceived by many patients. Patients are encouraged to delineate what they are responsible for in their lives and what is not under their control because of the disorder. The subsequent three monthly booster group sessions relive some of the issues discussed previously and provide an opportunity to integrate and implement many of the skills that were learned. In addition, they provide a forum to consider issues related to quality of life and long-term adjustment to their disease.

Didactic Group Therapy: Research Findings

Studies have shown that therapy groups that utilize psychoeducational and cognitive-behavioral approaches can be useful for patients suffering from non-bipolar depression (Kanas, 2000; Scott and Stradling, 1990; Shaffer et al., 1981; Thimm and Antonsen, 2014; Zettle, Haflich and Reynolds, 1992). But these approaches also have been useful for manic and depressive symptoms in bipolar patients.

Van Gent and Zwart (1993, 1994) developed a psychoeducational approach for treating bipolar patients combined with lithium prophylaxis. They followed 26 patients for nearly five years after they began ten sessions of psychoeducational group therapy. During the first five sessions, the patients were presented with information about their illness, lithium and its actions and side effects, and the consequences of stopping the medication. Although the primary emphasis was educational, elements from behavior therapy and Yalom's group techniques were included to keep the focus on present concerns. Patients were encouraged to share their feelings of anxiety about having a recurrence of mania or depression, its possible effect on their relatives, and personal experiences and solutions of dealing with an acute episode. The importance of recognizing prodromal symptoms also was discussed. In the last five sessions, discussion topics dealt with bipolar disorder as it pertained to leisure time, study, work, career, and financial issues. During the group treatment and for 15 months thereafter, self-esteem was reported as increased by 19 of the 26 patients, and subscale insufficiency in thinking and behaving on the psychoneurotic scale of the SCL-90 improved significantly. During the follow-up period, which averaged 51 months, episodes of discontinuing lithium decreased significantly from 24 before the group treatment to 12 at follow-up, and the number of readmissions to the hospital dropped from 21 to 8; both of these changes were significant.

Bauer and colleagues (1998) described a method of treating bipolar patients in group therapy with the goals of helping them manage their illness and improve their social and occupational functioning. The authors studied 29 VA outpatients who were diagnosed as having bipolar disorder and were assigned to therapy groups using a manualized treatment method constructed by the two senior authors. The groups meet weekly for 60 minutes and, typically, five to seven patients attended each session. Four therapists were trained to lead the groups, and their adherence to the manual was measured via audiotapes of the sessions. In Phase 1, the patients met for five weekly, structured psychoeducational sessions that focused on clinical aspects of bipolar disorder. Patients completed worksheets on their own specific patterns of illness and developed action plans that identified ways to cope with their symptoms. Phase 2 sessions were less structured, with patients identifying and dealing with various social and occupational problems resulting from their disorder. Worksheets and behaviorally measurable goals for improvement were incorporated into the discussions. Sixty-nine percent of the patients completed Phase 1, with the patients recording a significant improvement in a knowledge-based questionnaire pre- to post-group. In Phase 2, 70% of the patients had clear documentation of achieving at least one of their self-defined goals in social or occupational status. The therapists scored 90% or better on measures related to adherence to the manual, showing that the method could be taught reliably to group leaders.

In a series of papers, Weiss and his colleagues (1999, 2000, 2007) discussed and evaluated their group therapy method (which they called an "integrated" approach) for treating bipolar patients who also were diagnosed as having a substance-use disorder. They used a CBT model that was manual-based and consisted of 20 weekly hour-long meetings. It emphasized the similarities in thought and behavior patterns in recovery and relapse processes in the two disorders (Weiss et al., 1999, 2007). They first conducted a pilot study involving 45 dual-diagnosed patients, where they compared their approach to a no-group therapy control condition (where patients simply received six monthly assessments). They found that the group patients had significantly fewer days of drug use than those in the control condition (Weiss et al., 2000). They then conducted a randomized controlled study involving 62 dual-diagnosed patients to compare the effect of their group approach with an active treatment, group drug counseling, which also meet for 20 weekly hour-long meetings and was designed to approximate the treatment delivered in community substance abuse treatment programs (Weiss et al., 2007). Both groups were manual-based, with specific topics to be addressed. Bipolar and substance-use topics were both presented in the group using their approach, but only substance-use topics were presented in the drug counseling group. Overall, substance use decreased during treatment, but patients using their approach had significantly fewer days of substance use than the drug counseling patients, and usage remained lower during the three-month, post-treatment follow-up period. Most of the improvement was in alcohol use; drug use did not improve over time. Unexpectedly, there were more depressive and manic symptoms during treatment and follow-up for the group therapy patients than the drug counseling patients. Finally, group therapy patients attended significantly more group sessions than the drug counseling patients.

Patelis-Siotis and colleagues (2001) reported on the effectiveness of a 14-session, manualized group CBT treatment for medicated patients with bipolar disorder. The two-hour sessions were conducted weekly. Phase I (two sessions) focused on psychoeducation related to medications, symptoms, and course of the illness, and family members were included in the discussions of video and monograph material. Phase II was composed of 12 skill-training sessions that included specific behavioral and cognitive interventions from a treatment manual that targeted clinical features of bipolar disorder (both depression and mania), adherence to pharmacotherapy, and improvement of interpersonal issues related to coping with the consequence of this disease. Forty-nine patients were enrolled in the program, and 38 (78%) completed both phases of the group. The authors found that the patients showed significant improvement on measures of global psychosocial functioning and general medical outcome, especially on subscales measuring vitality and role-emotion. There was no improvement on measures of mood symptoms.

Colom et al. (2003b) have pointed out that poor adherence to treatment, especially pharmacotherapy, is common among bipolar patients and that this relates to their high rates of relapse. In addition, many of these patients relapse due to failure to recognize early signs of mania and depression, which could have been treated before escalating into a more serious episode. They developed a group therapeutic approach for bipolar patients that focused on educating them about the value of medications and recognizing early prodromal symptoms of their disease, such as hyperactivity and reduced need for sleep. The authors reported the results of a randomized single-blind study they conducted using 50 bipolar I patients, where all patients received standard psychiatric care and pharmacological treatment. Half of the patients were randomly assigned to participate in 20 weekly, nonspecific support groups (control condition), whereas the other half participated in 20 weekly, psychoeducational groups (experimental condition). The 90-minute experimental group sessions focused on four main issues: illness awareness, treatment compliance, early detection of prodromal symptoms and recurrences, and lifestyle regularity. These were addressed via an educational presentation by the group leader on the topic for that day, followed by a related in-group exercise and general discussion. The patients were studied during the group treatments and in a follow-up period of two years, during which time they only received the standard treatment. The results showed that the educational group patients as compared with the supportive group patients experienced significantly fewer recurrences of their illness and significantly fewer hospitalizations, both during the active treatment phase and in the two-year follow-up period. There were no significant differences regarding pharmacological treatment or mood-stabilizing blood levels. The authors believe that the early detection of prodromal symptoms played a central role in reducing the likelihood of recurrence.

Colom and his colleagues (2003a) extended their previous work (Colom et al., 2003b) to include 120 bipolar I and II outpatients who received standard psychiatric care and pharmacological treatment. As in their earlier report, half of the subjects were randomized to participate in 20 weekly, nonspecific support groups, and half (who were matched for age and sex) received 20 weekly, psychoeducational groups that focused on illness awareness, treatment compliance, early detection of prodromal symptoms and recurrences, and lifestyle regularity. Compared to the support group patients, the psychoeducational patients had significantly fewer relapses during both the group treatment period and during the two-year follow-up period, where the subjects just received medications. At 12, 18, and 24 months after treatment, the cumulative mean number of hospitalizations per patient was significantly lower for the psychoeducational patients, as was the mean number of days of hospitalization per patient. In addition, the time to depression, manic, hypomanic, and mixed recurrences was increased in the psychoeducational patients.

Goldner-Vukov, Moore and Cupina (2007) treated ten bipolar patients in a therapy group that focused on psychoeducational, cognitive, and existential issues. Sessions were held weekly for two hours over three months and then monthly for up to two years. During this time, two members had minor relapses that did not require hospitalization. All of the patients followed their pharmacotherapy regimen, and all reported improvements in family and social functioning. Nine patients remained employed in full-time jobs. Patients reported being very satisfied with the group approach.

In Chapter 3, I reported on the paper by Segredou et al. (2011), who conducted a review of group therapy studies from 1986 to mid-2006 that involved patients suffering from schizophrenia or bipolar disorder, had at least 20 participants, and included a control group (usually treatment as usual (TAU) or a waiting list). In all of the studies, there was significant improvement in the treatment condition in at least one important parameter. In the bipolar sample, all four studies that were reported used psychoeducational interventions and gave positive results; none used CBT or psychodynamic techniques.

Rahmani and colleagues (2016) conducted a randomized controlled study in Iran of 76 female bipolar inpatients who were randomly assigned to receive either TAU or TAU plus group therapy, which consisted of ten continuous, 90-minute, biweekly psychoeducation sessions. The group program emphasized the course and treatment of bipolar disorder, especially the importance of taking medications as prescribed in improving symptoms and preventing relapses. On two measures of medication adherence (a medicine check list and a medication adherence rating scale), there were no significant differences between the no-group and group patients prior to the group intervention. However, after the study intervention, the mean scores on both medication adherence measures were significantly higher in the group therapy patients than in the control patients. The authors concluded that "group psychoeducation seems an effective intervention for enhancing of medication adherence in pharmacologically treated patients with bipolar disorders" (p. 294).

Combined Treatment Approaches

In Chapter 2, I discussed the value of combining treatment approaches for schizophrenia spectrum patients. Similar attempts have been made to combine treatment approaches for bipolar patients. For example, the model presented by Cook et al. (2014) that blends educational and process-oriented approaches that was discussed in Chapter 2 also has relevance for people suffering from bipolar disorders. This Process-Oriented Psychoeducational (POP) group format encourages patients to interact, thus reducing isolation and enhancing cohesion, while at the same time teaching them about their illness and its warning signs and ways to cope with its symptoms. In defending their clinical approach, and based on their review of the literature, the authors concluded:

> Research in the treatment of bipolar disorder has suggested that process-oriented therapy encouraging the use of interpersonal skills, receiving feedback, self-awareness, and the emergence of therapeutic group factors can improve executive and overall functioning...In addition, psychoeducation can increase self-confidence, social functioning, and self-management abilities, leading to fewer relapses and hospitalizations for those with bipolar disorder.
>
> (Cook et al., 2014, pp. 186–187)

See Chapter 2 for details on this clinical approach.

Bouwkamp et al. (2013) have described a semi-structured behavioral and interpersonal form of group therapy for bipolar patients that they have called Interpersonal and Social Rhythm Therapy (IPSRT). The authors take the position that episodes of mania or depression are preceded by factors such as non-compliance with pharmacotherapy, stressful life events, or a disruption in social rhythms. The focus of IPSRT is to improve acceptance of the disease, increase compliance with mood-stabilizing medications, enhance healthy coping strategies with life pressures, and restore disrupted circadian rhythms (e.g., sleep/wake cycle, appetite, level of activity). Patients first participate in a Social Rhythm Therapy group consisting of 1½-hour weekly group sessions, where they are taught to use a Social Rhythm Metric (SRM) that measures five daily social events: time out of bed, time of first social interaction, time of start of daily activities, time of evening meal, and time to bed. Each week, the patients' daily SRM scores are discussed, and advice is given on ways they can stabilize their social rhythms. This is followed by the IPSRT group itself, which consists of 16 weekly sessions of two hours each: one hour that continues training in SRM, and one hour that focuses on interpersonal psychotherapy (IPT). The goals of the IPT component are to reduce mood symptoms and improve social and interpersonal relationships. Patients are asked to identify interpersonal problem areas and construct sociograms of their key relationships. They also are asked to record specific interpersonal events and accompanying mood states that occurred during the past week. These are discussed during the sessions. Group here-and-now interactions may be used to explore these problems further. The authors conducted a pre–post study of this group format and reported that SRM scores and a measure of depression significantly improved in 22 patients who completed treatment. There was no significant improvement in mania scores. In addition, the number of months depressed in the year post-treatment was significantly decreased as compared to the year before treatment.

Integrative Group Therapy for Non-Psychotic Bipolar Patients: Clinical Issues

As was the case for psychotic patients (see Chapter 4), an *integrative* group treatment model may be used for non-psychotic bipolar patients, which again is defined as *an evidence-based, group therapeutic approach that uses clinical principles that combine both non-didactic (psychodynamic and interpersonal) and didactic (psychoeducational and cognitive-behavioral) techniques into one coordinated treatment model.* But there are differences in emphasis between bipolar and psychosis groups.

Group Goals

Important treatment goals in conducting therapy groups with non-psychotic bipolar patients are listed in Table 7.1. Early in the life of the group, it is useful for the therapist to make presentations that educate the patients about the disorder: its genetics, typical course, and precipitating factors. Although familial and constitutional factors play a role in precipitating a depressive or manic episode, life stressors also are important (Swendsen et al., 1995), and patients need to identify school, work, and familial pressures in their lives that produce stress. The vulnerability-stress model discussed in Chapter 2 and the "U" curve external stimulation-symptom relationship illustrated in Vignette 4.9, Chapter 4, can be

Table 7.1 Goals of integrative group therapy for non-psychotic bipolar patients

Learn about the disorder: genetics, course, precipitating factors
Learn about the value of taking mood-stabilizing medications as prescribed
Recognize prodromal symptoms and coping actions to take to prevent an
   acute episode
Challenge distorted cognitions: despair of depression, exuberance of mania
Discuss important psychodynamic issues: dependency, pressure to achieve,
   denial, maladaptive personality traits
Learn ways to relate better with others through the here-and-now of the group

presented to bipolar patients as a way of thinking about the interplay of external stressors and constitutional factors on a person's emotional state. Following a presentation, ample time should be set aside for patients to discuss how what they were taught applies specifically to them, and they should share strategies of coping. Some therapists may invite significant others to attend these early sessions, so that everyone is on the same page as to the nature of the patient's bipolar disorder.

Information about mood-stabilizing medications and the need for compliance also may be presented formally to the patients early in the life of the group. As discussed earlier, poor compliance with mood-stabilizing medications is a relatively common occurrence among bipolar patients, and it increases the frequency of future manic and depressive episodes. Consequently, the group leader should present clinical and empirical information regarding this issue and encourage the patients to become conscious of times when such compliance issues have led them to develop an acute episode. Reasons for avoiding full compliance with prescribed medications should be discussed in the group as well, such as "I felt good, so I didn't think I needed to keep taking my medications" or "the medications slowed me down, and I could not be as productive as I wanted to be." Many bipolar patients are intelligent people who work in jobs that have high expectations that may be sustained by hypomanic work behavior. Returning to a more euthymic state may mean adjustments to their lifestyle, and they may be reluctant to make these changes. The alternative is a decompensation, which interferes more with productivity over a lifetime than lowering the energy level to a more modest pace. Such issues are best handled through group discussions, where the members can share feelings and gain support from others who are in the same situation.

Learning to recognize prodromal symptoms of an impending acute phase of illness is important, since coping actions sometimes can be taken to ameliorate the severity of a decompensation. Harbingers of an acute episode include factors such as disturbances in sleep or appetite, more frequent or intense mood swings, and feelings of despondency or irritability with others. Discriminating between what might be a "normal" emotional reaction to a life event and what might be an "abnormal" escalation toward mania or depression is very important. Although common prodromal symptoms can be presented by the group leader, there is individual variation between patients. Hence, it is important for group members to identify and share their unique vulnerabilities with each other during the group discussions. Likewise, coping strategies may be general (e.g., alerting a therapist, increasing the medication dose, avoiding stressors) or specific to a given person. For example, if dealing with a difficult relative raises a bipolar person's stress level, and if such stress seems to predict a manic or depressive episode, then avoiding the relative or learning behavioral strategies of reducing the stress he or she causes (e.g., relaxation training, meditation) might be useful prophylactically to prevent an acute decompensation.

Along these lines, common cognitive distortions of bipolar patients can be identified, such as the tendency of people who are depressed to feel despair and believe that they are the worst people on Earth, and those who are hypomanic to feel exuberant and believe that they can conquer the universe. Resulting behaviors include withdrawal and aggressive behavior. The A–B–C model discussed in Chapter 2 can be presented in bipolar groups, and alternative cognitions and behaviors can be explored through the use of member-to-member discussions, group exercises, and homework assignments.

As patients begin to bond and trust one another in the group, they are ready to discuss important psychodynamic themes found in many bipolar patients, such as strong dependency needs and pressure to achieve. Sharing such feelings with one another may help the group members realize that they are not alone. Sometimes, important insights occur that lead to conflict resolution and behavioral change. For example, a tendency in many bipolar patients to deny negative feelings of inferiority and replace them with aggressive behavior can be explored in the group with "tough love" and support, and alternate ways of thinking and behaving may result.

Finally, as discussed earlier, many bipolar patients have problems relating well with other people, despite superficial conformity and sociability. On the one hand, they may be isolative and avoidant; on the other hand, hypercompetitive and aggressive. Some of these characteristics are embedded in their personalities. Indeed, maladaptive personality traits and even diagnosable personality disorders are commonly found in bipolar patients (Merikangas et al., 2007; Volkmar et al., 1981). Since these characteristics have interpersonal sequelae, they can be dealt with in the here-and-now of the group, since such maladaptive interactions can be observed and discussed in real time during the sessions.

Discussion Topics

These goals lend themselves to a number of discussion topics. Some examples are shown in Table 7.2. Sometimes, the therapist will introduce an agenda item for that day, such as presenting information about the disorder or medications, or introducing a new group member and saying goodbye to a departing member or cotherapist (see Chapter 4). When formal homework has been assigned, or when a topic was introduced late in the previous session without adequate discussion, the therapist may refer to these issues in the subsequent meeting.

Cerbone et al. (1992) and Hallensleben (1994) have found that early in the life of closed outpatient bipolar groups, learning about the disorder,

Table 7.2 Discussion topics in integrative group therapy for non-psychotic bipolar patients

Characteristics of bipolar disorder
Effects and side effects of mood-stabilizing medications
Resistance to taking medications as prescribed
Prodromal symptoms of manic and depressive episodes
Distorted cognitions about the self during mania and depression
Dependency and counter-dependency
Use of denial and possible underlying personality disorder
Pressure to conform and achieve
Frustration that episodes interfere with life goals (e.g., work, school, family)
Inability to control one's own emotional state
Despair over having a chronic mental illness
Potential for suicide
Interpersonal ramifications of the disorder

issues involving proper medication use, supporting one another, and establishing cohesion and camaraderie dominate the sessions. I have found the same early characteristics in the integrative group approach, although I would add consideration of prodromal symptoms as another topic that is appropriate for early group discussions.

Later on, as the members become more comfortable with each other, psychodynamic and interpersonal issues will be more likely to be discussed. Like in the psychosis groups, sessions might begin with silence from the leader or priming question such as: "How is everyone today?" or "How has your week gone?" Ideally, patients will spontaneously raise an issue related to some topic mentioned in Table 7.2. Like in psychosis groups, there are two reasons for this open-ended beginning. First, if a patient has a burning issue to discuss, he or she would be free to bring it up without blockage by a therapist's agenda item. Second, it reinforces that the group belongs to the members and that they share responsibility for its content. If the members bring up an issue seemingly unrelated to their bipolar disorder, the therapist might point this out and ask the patients to share the relevance of the topic to the goals of the group. Since most patients in bipolar groups are free of current psychosis, the groups can be managed with less structure and direction that is the case for patients in psychosis groups.

Clinical Illustration of a Typical Session

The setting was an outpatient bipolar group with seven patients and two psychiatrist coleaders (a staff member supervisor, Dr. K, and a resident trainee). It had been meeting for several weeks. The session began with a general discussion brought up by the patients of medication side effects and the need to take mood-stabilizing medications as prescribed to deal with bipolar disorders. Peter said that despite taking medications, he experienced brief episodes of depression during the two years following his last manic episode and that this seemed to be a baseline state for him. Dr. K asked if other group members had similar experiences. Some patients said that they felt either a little low or a little high some of the time, whereas the rest of the patients said that they felt emotionally more in the middle.

Sam went on to describe feeling depressed and hopeless pretty continuously over the past several months. He wondered if this might not be a warning of an impending depressed episode, although he had no other symptoms or signs that suggested this. As he spoke, Dr. K observed that Sam spoke in a complaining manner, with a fair amount of energy. Oscar tried to console Sam by suggesting that he might gain more purpose in life and elevate his spirits by doing volunteer work. Sam lashed back, saying that this wouldn't work, since his bipolar condition prevented him from keeping a paid job. He even had been "fired" from a previous volunteer activity. When other group members further tried to console Sam, he repeatedly and angrily rejected their input. He seemed intent on convincing the other group members that he was worthless, but at the same time he seemed to be disparaging the other members' suggestions while monopolizing the discussion.

Dr. K commented on Sam's rejecting comments and wondered if his responses were more of a personality "thing" than a manifestation of his bipolar disorder. Dr. K further suggested that this behavior might be related to his problems finding and keeping employment. Although Sam denied this linkage, he seemed thoughtful of Dr. K's comments. This led to a general discussion in the group of personality traits versus symptoms of mania and depression, and how difficult it was at times to tell the difference.

In this session, several notable events occurred. First, the group engaged in a discussion of mood-stabilizers and the importance of taking these medications as prescribed, echoing information they had been presented by the leader in an earlier session. Second, Sam began to wonder if his depressed mood over the past several months might be a warning of an impending depressive episode, another topic presented in an earlier session. But the length of time and stability of his mood, the absence of other symptoms, and his resistive response to feedback from other group members led Dr. K to suspect that his dysphoria was related more to his personality than to an upcoming depressed episode. He commented on this possibility, and although Sam was somewhat resistive to this interpretation, it led to a discussion in the group about the relationship between personality traits and an overlying bipolar disorder.

Differences From Integrative Psychosis Groups

The treatment of patients with schizophrenia spectrum and other psychotic disorders that was discussed in previous chapters also employs an integrative approach. However, there are differences in approach between these psychosis groups and non-psychosis bipolar groups, and these are listed in Table 7.3. Note that some of these differences are just a matter of emphasis and should be viewed simply as guidelines for the clinician.

Obviously, coping with psychotic symptoms is not part of non-psychosis bipolar groups. Bipolar patients who want to discuss previous or current lingering psychotic symptoms and signs are referred to the psychosis group. Information about the illness and its course is not given great emphasis in psychosis groups, but it is in bipolar groups, even to the point of formal presentations made by the group leader. The same goes for medication effects and dosage. Difficulty coping with side effects may be considered in either treatment model, as are compliance issues, but the latter is given more time in the bipolar group. Prodromal symptoms, signaling an impending acute exacerbation, are given more emphasis in the bipolar group, since they often consist of subtle mood and sleep changes that patients may miss or confuse with normal variations in their circadian cycle. In the psychosis group, topics related to important

Table 7.3 Differences between integrative psychosis groups and non-psychosis bipolar groups

Integrative psychosis group	Integrative non-psychosis bipolar group
Major goal is coping with psychotic symptoms (hallucinations, delusions, loose associations)	Coping with psychotic symptoms rarely discussed (psychotic patients are referred to psychosis group)
Formal presentations about the disorder sometimes done by the group leader	Formal presentations about the disorder commonly done by the group leader
Characteristics of antipsychotic medications sometimes discussed	Characteristics of mood-stabilizing medications commonly discussed, especially compliance issues
Recognizing prodromal symptoms sometimes discussed	Recognizing prodromal symptoms commonly discussed
Psychodynamic themes are discussed only later in stable mature groups (typically, after four to six months)	Psychodynamic themes commonly considered (e.g., dependency, denial, long-term psychological/personality problems)
Interpersonal issues are commonly considered, using the here-and-now to illustrate points	Interpersonal issues are commonly considered, using the here-and-now to illustrate points
Leader active and monitors the group process to keep the patients on track	Leader less active and gives the patients more leeway in the group process to go where they want

psychodynamic themes (e.g., long-standing problems contributing to the symptoms of the disorder, maladaptive patterns of relating with others) are considered only after some four to six months, when the members have bonded together. Even then, the therapist is cautious about the degree of uncovering, regression, and affect expression that occurs. The uncovering of relevant psychodynamic issues such as dependency and denial is more typically a part of non-psychosis bipolar groups, partly because of their common occurrence and partly because euthymic bipolar patients are better able to tolerate the emotions that result from these discussions. Interpersonal issues are discussed in both integrated psychosis and bipolar groups, and the here-and-now interactions of the members are used to illustrate important interpersonal clinical points. Finally, the leader is more active and monitors the group process to keep the patients on track in psychosis groups, whereas he or she allows the members more leeway to develop topics and interact with each other spontaneously in bipolar groups (which they sometimes do with great energy!).

Patient Inclusion or Exclusion

Bipolar therapy groups are for patients who have experienced manic and depressive episodes and currently are euthymic and able to meet the demands of group therapy (e.g., show some psychological-mindedness, be able to respond to therapeutic input, interact with other people). Mildly depressed and hypomanic patients usually can tolerate the group experience as well.

Bipolar groups are not for patients who are acutely psychotic or who have severe coexisting substance abuse (but see the special group format developed by Weiss et al. [1999, 2000, 2007], discussed earlier). Severely depressed patients who are withdrawn to the point of being unresponsive generally make poor group members. Group therapy also is not indicated for patients who are in an acute manic phase, since the stimulation of receiving multiple interpersonal inputs may escalate their symptoms and lead to further decompensation. Patients with manic symptoms also can be a challenge for the other group members, as can be seen in the following clinical vignette:

> Vignette 7.1. Patient A, a member in an ongoing outpatient bipolar group, regressed into a minor manic episode. He frequently came late, dominated the sessions with extraneous questions about the group format, and once even appeared in a werewolf mask! This group was being monitored as part of a research study (Kanas and Cox, 1998), and group scores on an anxiety/tension measure were very high during these sessions, even though the mean scores otherwise were very low. The group also experienced a transient drop in attendance. In fact, A's own attendance declined until he could be adequately treated with medication and return in a more stable condition.

Group Format

The format issues shown in Table 4.5 for integrative psychosis groups generally hold true for integrative bipolar groups, except that the latter can meet for a minimum of 60 minutes, and the number of patients included in the inpatient setting can be higher (see Table 7.4). Inpatient bipolar groups likely will occur only on specialized units for mood disorders, where there are a large number of potential patients. In most inpatient settings, stable bipolar patients likely will be mixed in with other non-psychotic group patients.

Group Process

Like in many therapy groups involving non-psychotic patients, bipolar therapy groups that are closed to new admissions would be expected to go through a series of sequential stages, although this issue needs to be studied further. In open groups with frequent patient turnover, there usually is a regression toward earlier themes and ways of behaving until the new members are brought up to the same level of comfort and trust as the members who have been in the group longer. This "new" group then moves forward in terms of cohesion and ability to discuss intimate topics.

Although outwardly functional in many ways, euthymic bipolar patients suffer from two important clinical problems (other than their potential for acute manic and depressive episodes). First, as mentioned above, they have a high incidence of personality disorders, making them somewhat resistive to psychotherapy. Second, they have difficulty modulating emotional states and may react with emotional fragility in the group, such as excessive cynicism and proneness to despondency, or excessive euphoria and high energy. Therefore, therapists conducting integrative bipolar therapy groups need to accommodate these tendencies. For example, when addressing a patient about his anger at another patient in the group, if the therapist is too confrontive, he or she may be met with denial, depression, or hypomania, so some sensitivity is indicated.

Table 7.4 Group format issues: non-psychosis bipolar groups

Issue	Inpatient groups	Outpatient groups
Sessions per week	3–5	1–2
Duration of session	60 minutes	60–90 minutes
Type of group	Open	Closed or slow-open
Number of therapists	2	1–2
Enrolled patients	6–9	6–10
Ideal number of patients in a session	5–7	6–8

In other cases, life events beyond the control of the group may trigger strong emotions, as the following vignette illustrates:

> Vignette 7.2. Patient B, enrolled in a VA outpatient bipolar group, was an accomplished film-maker who chronically had a high energy level and several ongoing projects. He especially was proud of a recent documentary that was shown on a national television station. His latest project was buying an old movie theater in his community and converting it into a larger complex, complete with retail shopping and other amenities. But getting financial backing for this project was very difficult, and he was becoming more and more anxious and frustrated. The group leader and several of the group members tried to convince him to scale back on this project to one that was more realistic and took less of a toll on him emotionally, but he denied the extent of his problems and ignored the feedback. Over time, he started to believe he would fail, and indeed he got himself into financial difficulties. This resulted in his becoming depressed, which decreased his energy level and led to further frustration. He subsequently stopped coming to group despite attempts to retain him. Several months later, he committed suicide.

This patient's success was built on his skills and energetic life style. When he met a challenge beyond his reach, he avoided the group's feedback and persisted nevertheless, since this had worked for him before in his various projects. He ultimately dropped out of treatment and ended his life.

Some patients have difficulty understanding whether an emotional high or low represents a transient mood variation or signals the beginning of a manic or depressive decompensation. Other patients experience fear and despair over the destructive impact that future mood swings may have in their vocational and interpersonal life. Thus, emotional themes are paramount in non-psychotic bipolar groups.

In Chapter 2, I considered the therapeutic factor model originally developed by Yalom (1970, 1975). Using this system, Shakir et al. (1979) listed interpersonal learning, instillation of hope, and imparting of information as three therapeutic factors that they observed in their bipolar group. Kripke and Robinson (1985) concluded that seven of Yalom's therapeutic factors operated in their group: imparting of information, installation of hope, universality, altruism, imitative behavior, interpersonal learning, and group cohesiveness. Pollack (1990) believed that the goal of sharing information in her inpatient group could be achieved by the therapeutic factor of imparting information; the goal of learning to cope with their illness could be achieved by universality, instillation of hope, group cohesiveness, and altruism; and the goal of improving interpersonal relationships could be achieved by the therapeutic factors of interpersonal learning and development of socialization techniques. Thus, it appears that the kinds of therapeutic factors Yalom found to be operative in his groups of patients with neurotic and personality problems also can be observed in groups with bipolar patients.

Therapist Stance

Bipolar patients can be very challenging and take their toll on therapists. Cohen et al. (1954) have pointed out two important transference issues in dealing with bipolar patients in group therapy: their clinging dependency and their stereotyped approach to others. Sometimes, they use people for their own needs in an exploitative manner, and these traits arouse strong countertransference feelings of anger and frustration in some therapists, or they may view demanding and extroverted bipolar patients as superficial and uninteresting (Winther, 1994). In dealing with bipolar patients, the therapist needs to set firm limits, engage them at an emotional level, avoid being seduced by outward attempts at friendship, focus on rational issues, and be aware of their own strong countertransference feelings. So, in addition to some of the factors supporting cotherapy in groups discussed in Chapter 4, the countertransference implication of treating bipolar patients in groups adds another reason to have two therapists in attendance who can discuss such feelings in their post-session rehashes.

Effectiveness of the Integrative Model for Non-Psychotic Bipolar Patients

Kanas and Cox (1998) evaluated group process during the first 31 sessions of a bipolar therapy group at the mental health outpatient clinic of the San Francisco Department of Veterans Affairs Medical Center (SFVA). The group met for 75-minute weekly sessions and was studied during the first seven months of its existence. There were two trained cotherapists, a staff psychiatrist and a psychiatric resident. Overall, 12 patients participated in the group, all of whom were euthymic or mildly hypomanic or depressed. Each patient attended an average of 10.7 sessions, and the attendance rate was 72%. After each session, the therapists evaluated the group process using the short form of MacKenzie's Group Climate Questionnaire (MacKenzie, 1983, 1990; MacKenzie and Livesley, 1983). Three major dimensions were scored—Engagement, Avoidance, and Conflict—as well as a scale measuring the degree of anxiety/tension. Also after each session, the therapists wrote down the most important topics that were discussed. At the end of the study, the topics were placed in one of five categories. Three were related to the goals of the group (i.e., learning more about bipolar disorder and mood-stabilizing medications; discussing strategies of coping with the symptoms of the disease; and uncovering important psychodynamic and interpersonal issues associated with bipolar disorder, such as the role of personality traits, denial, and maladaptive relationships with others). A fourth category dealt with general group issues, such as introducing new members to the group and discussions of attendance, and the last category was for miscellaneous other topics.

Using t-tests, the overall mean score of the bipolar group on the Engaged dimension was significantly higher compared with the overall mean score for MacKenzie's (1983) normative group sample. In contrast, the bipolar patient mean scores were significantly lower on the Avoiding and Conflict dimensions. Although MacKenzie did not report scores for his anxiety/tension scale, the overall mean score of 1.58 translated to a rating of between "a little bit" and "somewhat." The therapists also compared the bipolar group scores to the overall mean scores on one of the integrative long-term outpatient psychosis therapy groups composed largely of schizophrenic patients (Kanas, DiLella and Jones, 1984)—see Table 6.3, column 4. The results were the same: bipolar group patients scored significantly higher in Engaged and significantly lower in Avoiding, Conflict, and anxiety/tension.

The analysis of the 103 discussion topics revealed that 40% were placed in the coping with symptoms category, 30% were in the disorder-related psychodynamic or interpersonal issue category, 18% were placed in the general group issues category, 11% were in the learning more about the disease and its medical management category, and 1% were in the miscellaneous category (i.e., a discussion of a lost wallet and what to do about it).

The high Engaged score suggested that the patients in this bipolar group were very cohesive and able to relate well with each other compared to other therapy groups. The low Avoiding, Conflict and anxiety/tension scores suggested that the patients felt free to discuss their issues openly in an atmosphere that was relatively free of interpersonal friction and anxiety. The analysis of the discussion topics suggested that the group members discussed issues appropriate to their needs: 81% of the topics were related to one of the three group goals, especially coping with their disorder and discussions related to relevant psychodynamic and interpersonal issues. Notably, most of the 11% of the topics that related to information about bipolar disorder and its medical management occurred when the group began and whenever new patients were admitted. "It was as if these more factual discussions served to orient new members into the group until they became able to discuss more psychologically painful topics later on." (Kanas and Cox, 1998, p. 43).

Graves (1993) reported on his experience with a therapy group for 14 bipolar patients that met over the course of nine years, during which time there were three complete turnovers of the group population. The average time spent in the group per patient was 2.9 years. His treatment approach was intermediate between Yalom's higher-level focus group (Yalom, 1983) and a more open-ended, process-oriented outpatient group method that included my integrative model for schizophrenic patients (Kanas, 1985). The focus was on adaptive functioning to bipolar illness using a here-and-now, reality-based orientation. The majority of the patients were people with bipolar disorder and a concomitant diagnosis of a "character" (i.e., personality) disorder. Themes and stages of recovery included: manic disorganization/depressive withdrawal, acute loss of self-esteem, reorganization and reconstruction during symptom-free periods, hypomanic breakthrough with bargaining and testing, and working through to a new identity.

Graves reported that prior to entering the group, the patients averaged 0.97 episodes of hospitalization per year, but that during their group involvement, this dropped to 0.18 episodes per year. Nine patients had depressive or manic regressions, which they felt would have led to hospitalization had they not had the support of the group members. Graves attributed this successful group outcome to three factors: increased medication compliance, decreased denial regarding the illness, and increased awareness of both external and internal stress factors leading to episodes.

Gonzalez and Prihoda (2007) conducted a controlled study of a long-duration outpatient group for bipolar patients. They described their approach as using "psychoeducation regarding illness, illness management, and exploration of dynamic and interpersonal issues" (p. 405). They further stated that they "adapted the Integrative Outpatient Model (IOM), developed by Nick Kanas for bipolar disorder" (p. 407). Eleven outpatients with bipolar disorder were assigned to receive TAU plus an outpatient therapy group that met in 90-minute weekly sessions for 16 months and then biweekly for two months. The first five sessions of the group consisted of formal psychoeducation presentations concerning bipolar disorder and medication adherence based on an agenda for each session. The remaining sessions consisted of the less-structured IOM approach, where the content for each session was not predetermined. Discussions reflected group member interests and ranged from education and illness management of bipolar disorder and medication effects and side effects to relevant psychodynamic themes and interpersonal issues. Their outcome was compared to 11 matched bipolar outpatients who were assigned for the same period of time to a TAU-only control condition.

All patients in the Gonzalez and Prihoda study were assessed at baseline, 18 months, and one year later using a variety of global functioning, mood symptom, and clinical status measures as well as the number of days per week they were "well" (i.e., recovered or subsyndromal). The drop-out rate for the group patients was 27%. Comparing the one-year follow-up assessment to the termination assessment, group patients were significantly less likely to be in a mood episode and had fewer depressive symptoms than the control patients. There were no significant between-group differences in manic symptoms or global assessment of functioning. The number of days "well" per week was significantly higher at the end of treatment and throughout the one-year follow-up period for the group patients, but there were no changes during the same time intervals for the controls.

These research studies involving the integrative approach for non-psychosis bipolar therapy groups generally have supported this treatment model. The patients have been able to interact productively, discuss a number of intrapsychic and interpersonal issues that are pertinent to their bipolar disorder, and support one another during hypomanic and depressive episodes.

References

Ablon, S.L., Davenport, Y.B., Gershon, E.S. and Adland, M.L. (1975) The married manic. *American Journal of Orthopsychiatry*, 45, 854–866.

American Psychiatric Association. (2013) *Diagnostic and Statistical Manual of Mental Disorders, Fifth Edition (DSM-5)*. Washington, D.C.: American Psychiatric Publishing.

Bauer, M.S., McBride, L., Chase, C., Sachs, G. and Shea, N. (1998) Manual-based group psychotherapy for bipolar disorder: A feasibility study. *Journal of Clinical Psychiatry*, 59, 449–455.

Bieling, P.J., McCabe, R.E. and Antony, M.M. (2009) Bipolar disorder. In: P.J. Bieling, R.E. McCabe and M.M. Antony (Eds.), *Cognitive-Behavioral Therapy in Groups*. New York: Guilford Press, pp. 239–265.

Bouwkamp, C.G., De Kruiff, M.E., Van Troost, T.M., Snippe, D., Blom, M.J., De Winter, R.F.P. and Haffmans, P.M.J. (2013) Interpersonal and social rhythm group therapy for patients with bipolar disorder. *International Journal of Group Psychotherapy*, 63, 97–114.

Cerbone, M.J.A., Mayo, J.A., Cuthbertson, B.A. and O'Connell, R.A. (1992) Group therapy as an adjunct to medication in the management of bipolar affective disorder. *Group*, 16(3), 174–187.

Cohen, M.B., Baker, G., Cohen, R.A., Fromm-Reichmann, F. and Weigert, E.V. (1954) An intensive study of twelve cases of manic-depressive psychosis. *Psychiatry*, 17, 103–137.

Colom, F., Vieta, E., Martinez-Aran, A., Reinares, M., Goikolea, J.M., Benabarre, A., … Corominas, J. (2003a) A randomized trial on the efficacy of group psychoeducation in the prophylaxis of recurrences in bipolar patients whose disease in in remission. *Archives of General Psychiatry*, 60, 402–407.

Colom, F., Vieta, E., Reinares, M., Martinez-Aran, A., Torrent, C., Goikolea, J.M., and Gasto, C. (2003b) Psychoeducation efficacy in bipolar disorders: Beyond compliance enhancement. *Journal of Clinical Psychiatry*, 64, 1101–1105.

Cook, W.G., Arechiga, A., Dobson, L.A. and Boyd K. (2014) Brief heterogeneous inpatient psychotherapy groups: A process-oriented psychoeducational (POP) model. *International Journal of Group Psychotherapy*, 64, 181–206.

Davenport, Y.B., Ebert, M.H., Adland, M.L. and Goodwin, F.K. (1977) Couples group therapy as an adjunct to lithium management of the manic patient. *American Journal of Orthopsychiatry*, 47, 495–502.

Gibson, R.W. (1958) The family background and early life experience of the manic-depressive patient. *Psychiatry*, 21, 71–90.

Gibson, R.W., Cohen, M.B. and Cohen, R.A. (1959) On the dynamics of the manic-depressive personality. *American Journal of* Psychiatry, 115, 1101–1107.

Goldner-Vukov, M., Moore, L.J. and Cupina, D. (2007) Bipolar disorder: From psychoeducational to existential group therapy. *Australasian Psychiatry*, 15(1), 30–34.

Gonzalez, J.M. and Prihoda, T.J. (2007) A case study of psychodynamic group psychotherapy for bipolar disorder. *American Journal of Psychotherapy*, 61, 405–422.

Graves, J.S. (1993) Living with mania: A study of outpatient group psychotherapy for bipolar patients. *American Journal of Psychotherapy*, 47, 113–126.

Hallensleben, A. (1994) Group psychotherapy with manic-depressive patients on lithium: Ten years' experience. *Group Analysis*, 27, 475–482.

Janowsky, D.S., EI-Yousef, M.K. and Davis, J.M. (1974) Interpersonal maneuvers of manic patients. *American Journal of Psychiatry*, 131, 250–255.

Janowsky, D.S., Leff, M. and Epstein, R.S. (1970) Playing the manic game: Interpersonal maneuvers of the acutely manic patient. *Archives of General Psychiatry*, 22, 252–261.

Kanas, N. (1985) Inpatient and outpatient group therapy for schizophrenic patients. *American Journal of Psychotherapy*, 39, 431–439.

Kanas, N. (1993) Group psychotherapy with bipolar patients: A review and synthesis. *International Journal of Group Psychotherapy*, 43, 321–333.

Kanas, N. (2000) Cognitive-behavioral group therapy for depression. *International Journal of Group Psychotherapy*, 50, 413–416.

Kanas, N. and Cox, P. (1998) Process and content in a therapy group for bipolar outpatients. *Group*, 22(1), 37–42.

Kanas, N., DiLella, V.J. and Jones, J. (1984) Process and content in an outpatient schizophrenic group. *Group*, 8(2), 13–20.

Kaplan, H.I. and Sadock, B.J. (1989) *Comprehensive Textbook of Psychiatry*, 5th ed. Baltimore, MD: Williams & Wilkins.

Kripke, D.F. and Robinson, D. (1985) Ten years with a lithium group. *McLean Hospital Journal*, 10, 1–11.

MacKenzie, K.R. (1983) The clinical application of a group climate measure. In: R.R. Dies and K.R. Makenzie (Eds.), *Advances in Group Psychotherapy: Integrating Research and Practice*. New York: International Universities Press, pp. 159–170.

MacKenzie, K.R. (1990) *Introduction to Time-Limited Group Psychotherapy*. Washington, D.C.: American Psychiatric Press.

MacKenzie, K.R. and Livesley, W.J. (1983) A developmental model for brief group therapy. In: R.R. Dies and K.R. Makenzie (Eds.), *Advances in Group Psychotherapy: Integrating Research and Practice*. New York: International Universities Press, pp. 101–116.

Merikangas, K.R., Akiskal, H.S., Angst, J., Greenberg, P.E., Hirschfeld, R.M.A., Petukhova, M., and Kessler, R.C. (2007) Lifetime and 12-month prevalence of bipolar spectrum disorder in the National Comorbidity Survey Replication. *Archives of General Psychiatry*, 64, 543–552.

Merriam-Webster Medical Dictionary (sourced in 2019), https://www.merriam-webster.com/medical

O'Connell, R.A., Mayo, J.A., Eng, L.K., Jones, J.S. and Gable, R.H. (1985) Social support and long-term lithium outcome. *British Journal of Psychiatry*, 147, 272–275.

Palmer, A.G., Williams, H. and Adams, M. (1995) CBT in a group format for bipolar affective disorder. *Behavioural and Cognitive Psychotherapy*, 23, 153–168.

Patelis-Siotis, I., Young, L.T., Robb, J.C., Marriott, M., Bieling, P.J., Cox, L.C and Joffe, R.T. (2001) Group cognitive behavioral therapy for bipolar disorder: A feasibility and effectiveness study. *Journal of Affective Disorders*, 65, 145–153.

Pollack, L.E. (1990) Improving relationships: Groups for inpatients with bipolar disorder. *Journal of Psychosocial Nursing*, 28(5), 17–22.

Rahmani, F., Ebrahimi, H., Ranjbar, F., Razavi, S.S. and Asghari, E. (2016) The effect of group psychoeducation program on medication adherence in patients with bipolar mood disorders: A randomized controlled trial. *Journal of Caring Sciences*, 5(4), 287–297.

Sajatovic, M., Davies, M. and Hrouda, D.R. (2004) Enhancement of treatment adherence among patients with bipolar disorder. *Psychiatric Services*, 55, 264–269.

Scott, J. and Pope, M. (2002) Self-reported adherence to treatment with mood stabilizers, plasma levels, and psychiatric hospitalization. *American Journal of Psychiatry*, 159, 1927–1929.

Scott, M.J. and Stradling, S.G. (1990) Group cognitive therapy for depression produces clinically significant reliable change in community-based settings. *Behavioral and Cognitive Psychotherapy*, 18, 1–19.

Segredou, I., Xenitidis, K., Panagiotopoulou, M., Bochtsou, V., Antoniadou, O. and Livaditis, M. (2011) Group psychosocial interventions for adults with schizophrenia and bipolar illness: The evidence base in the light of publications between 1986 and 2006. *International Journal of Social Psychiatry*, 58, 229–238.

Shaffer, C.S., Shapiro, J., Sank, L.I. and Coghlan, D.J. (1981) Positive changes in depression, anxiety, and assertion following individual and group cognitive behavior therapy intervention. *Cognitive Therapy and Research*, 5(2), 149–157.

Shakir, S.A., Volkmar, F.R., Bacon, S. and Pfefferbaum, A. (1979) Group psychotherapy as an adjunct to lithium maintenance. *American Journal of Psychiatry*, 136, 455–456.

Swendsen, J., Hammen, C., Heller, T. and Gitlin, M. (1995) Correlates of stress reactivity in patients with bipolar disorder' *American Journal of Psychiatry*, 152, 795–797.

Thimm, J.C. and Antonsen, L. (2014) Effectiveness of cognitive behavioral group therapy for depression in routine practice. *BMC Psychiatry*, 14, 292.

Van Gent, E.M. and Zwart, F.M. (1993) Five year follow-up after educational group therapy added to lithium prophylaxis: Five years after group added to lithium. *Depression*, 1, 225–226.

Van Gent, E.M. and Zwart, F.M. (1994) A long follow-up after group therapy in conjunction with lithium prophylaxis. *Nordic Journal of Psychiatry*, 1, 9–12.

Volkmar, F.R., Bacon, S., Shakir, S.A. and Pfefferbaum, A. (1981) Group therapy in the management of manic-depressive illness. *American Journal of Psychiatry*, 35, 226–234.

Weiss, R.D., Najavits, L.M. and Greenfield, S.F. (1999) A relapse prevention group for patients with bipolar and substance use disorders. *Journal of Substance Abuse treatment*, 16, 47–54.

Weiss, R.D., Griffin, M.L., Greenfield, S.F., Najavits, L.M., Wyner, D., Soto, J.A. and Hennen, J.A. (2000) Group therapy for patients with bipolar disorder and substance dependence: Results of a pilot study. *Journal of Clinical Psychiatry*, 61, 361–367.

Weiss, R.D., Griffin, M.L., Kolodziej, M.E., Greenfield, S.F., Najavits, L.M., Daley, D.C., ... Hennen, J.A. (2007) A randomized trial of integrated group therapy versus group drug counseling for patients with bipolar disorder and substance dependence. *American Journal of Psychiatry*, 164, 100–107.

Winther, G. (1994) Psychotherapy with manic-depressives: Problems in interaction between patient and therapist. *Group Analysis*, 27, 467–474.

Wulsin, L., Bachop, M. and Hoffman, D. (1988) Group therapy in manic-depressive illness. *American Journal of Psychotherapy*, 42, 263–271.

Yalom, I.D. (1970) *The Theory and Practice of Group Psychotherapy*. New York: Basic Books.

Yalom, I.D. (1975) *The Theory and Practice of Group Psychotherapy*, 2nd ed. New York: Basic Books.

Yalom, I.D. (1983) *Inpatient Group Psychotherapy*. New York: Basic Books.

Zettle, R.D., Haflich, J.L. and Reynolds, R.A. (1992) Responsivity of cognitive therapy as a function of treatment format and client personality dimensions. *Journal of Clinical Psychology*, 48, 787–797.

8 Conclusions

Therapy groups have been used to treat psychotic patients since the early 1920s, when Edward Lazell first described a treatment approach that was based on psychoanalytic theory but used a lecture format coupled with group discussions. The goal was to help patients with dementia praecox, as schizophrenia then was called, to learn more about their disorder and ways to cope with it. Since then, approaches for treating psychotic patients in therapy groups have emerged from the psychoanalytic/psychodynamic, interpersonal, psychoeducational, and cognitive-behavioral (CBT) schools of thought. These approaches have been effective. Based on large reviews of controlled studies comparing treatment groups for psychotic patients with control conditions, 78% of groups using an interaction-oriented, interpersonal focus had a significant advantage, versus 80% of psychoeducational groups and 83% of CBT groups. Only groups using a psychoanalytic, insight-oriented focus scored lower: 36% of such groups were better than controls. In some of the groups using this focus, patients actually performed worse, but these were older studies that used more traditional techniques (e.g., free association, transference interpretations) aimed at uncovering anxiety-producing unconscious conflicts. More current psychodynamic models include more support and less uncovering.

Taken alone, each of these four approaches have continued to be used in therapy groups for psychotic patients; but in their pure forms, they have some disadvantages. Psychoeducation and CBT do not pay enough attention to the interpersonal needs of these isolated individuals, and the lecture format may not allow enough time for maladaptive interactions to be addressed. Also, the presence of a planned lecture sequence with predetermined agendas does not allow enough flexibility to deal with crises and topics that may be of special interest to the patients attending the group that day. Psychodynamic and interpersonal approaches are more flexible, since they are more open-ended and discussion-oriented, but if there is too much emphasis on techniques using insight and transference, unpleasant memories and affects may result. In addition, by focusing on the past, many psychoanalytic models do not pay enough attention to interpersonal interactions in the here-and-now of the group. The interpersonal approach does, but at the risk of short-changing issues related to coping with symptoms, strengthening important ego functions like reality sense and reality testing, and discussing psychological problems concerning non-relationship issues. Also, like too much uncovering, the here-and-now focus can at times be too intensive, particularly around affect expression.

An *integrative* approach is called for that borrows the best from these four schools of thought. Especially if it is empirically derived and supported by good clinical research, a treatment approach can be developed that meets the needs of psychotic patients. These needs range from gaining a better understanding of their disease and its vicissitudes, to learning strategies of coping with their symptoms, to becoming better able to sense and test reality, to experimenting with different cognitive and behavioral strategies, to improving their interpersonal relationships. It also would meet the needs of the managed care revolution that calls for the development of treatment modalities that are useful, cost-effective, and evidence-based.

The integrative model presented in this book is defined as *an evidence-based, group therapeutic approach that uses clinical principles that combine both non-didactic (psychodynamic and interpersonal) and didactic (psychoeducational and cognitive-behavioral) techniques into one coordinated treatment model.* The two major goals of the integrative approach are to help the group members: (1) learn strategies of sensing/ testing reality and coping with their symptoms (e.g., hallucinations, delusions, disorganized thinking/speech, negative symptoms) and (2) improve their interpersonal relationships, with a focus on how the members interact with each other in the here-and-now of the group as a microcosm of how they relate outside of the group. Although group leaders at times use formal presentations to give information on the disease process and some psychoeducational and CBT principles (e.g., A–B–C and vulnerability-stress models, "U" curve of the external stimulation-symptom relationship), most of the sessions are open-ended, with patients setting the agenda, provided it is relevant to the group goals. A typical session will progress from *identifying* the topic for the day, to *generalizing* it to make sure that most attendees can relate to the topic, to a general discussion of *coping* strategies. The leader (or coleaders when two are involved) is active in focusing the group discussions on the topic at hand and keeping the topic relevant to the patients' psychiatric needs. Nevertheless, the group members are encouraged to give each other feedback in the here-and-now of the sessions rather than receiving advice from the leader. Concomitant antipsychotic medications are encouraged and definitely help, but often they are not enough for complete recovery, and many psychotic patients do not take them or refuse them altogether due to their troubling side effects.

New patients are told that: *this is a group for people who have had nervous breakdowns—we discuss issues such as hearing voices, feeling suspicious, being confused, or having problems relating with other people.* These goals dominate the discussion topics early in the life of the group. In later sessions (typically after four to six months), important psychodynamic themes and patterns in the patients' lives that have led to a distorted sense of reality and interfered with their ability to relate better with others are considered, with relevance to their impact on psychotic symptoms and current functioning.

Studies of integrative groups generally have supported the value of this approach. In terms of *outcome*, psychotic inpatients have rated the integrative group experience as being helpful, and psychiatric staff have noted improvements in how these patients interact with others on the ward. In the outpatient setting, the integrative model has been used in both long-term and time-limited short-term formats. Attendance rates typically are in the 80%–90% range, and drop-out rates usually are under 20%. Psychotic patients have experienced symptom reduction, a lowering of social anxiety, and improvement in their relationships with others, and some of these improvements have continued for several months after concluding the group experience. The majority of patients who completed a 12-session integrative group chose to enter a repeaters group that was offered two years later.

In studies of the integrative group *process* in both inpatient and outpatient settings, the members were found to engage in high quality work, show low levels of avoidance and conflict, and discuss their problems with minimal resistance and anxiety. Outpatient integrative groups show a pattern of increased cohesion and decreased avoidance and conflict as time goes on. Within the first few months of treatment, psychotic patients value the integrative groups more as a place to learn strategies of interacting with others, testing reality, and coping with psychotic symptoms than as a place to develop insight and receive advice concerning their illness, medications, or economic situations. In one long-term group, however, valued therapeutic factors clustered a bit more toward learning about their disorder, relating better with others, and expressing emotions than coping with symptoms such as hallucinations and delusions which suggests that these patients had learned coping strategies early on in the group and later were prepared to discuss and gain insight into more emotional and interpersonal issues, much like long-term groups with non-psychotic patients. The therapists in integrative groups have been found to be active and successful in shaping the parameters of the group that were congruent with the group goals. Mental health trainees reliably can be taught the integrative group therapy model with the hope that they will become leaders of future groups.

Integrative groups for psychotic patients are cost-effective. Patients receive help for their symptoms and for their interpersonal problems, and attendance rates are high. Inpatients value their experience and become interested in participating in similar groups as outpatients, which improves their long-term clinical course. Even in cotherapy groups, the staff-to-patient ratio is cost-effective: 1:3 or 1:4. Participation in the groups obviates the need for more staff-intensive 1:1 individual therapy. Short-term groups that are based on the integrative model have been found to be safe and beneficial, and especially in the outpatient setting, they represent a less expensive alternative to long-term group therapy.

The integrative groups discussed above are for patients suffering from psychotic symptoms due to schizophrenia spectrum diagnoses (e.g., schizophrenia, schizoaffective disorder, delusional disorder) and unspecified chronic psychotic disorder. Also included is the occasional bipolar patient with lingering psychotic symptoms (e.g., tangential thoughts, grandiosity, irrational depressive despair). Bipolar patients in the acute manic phase of their disease are not candidates for any kind of group therapy, since the increased stimulation can make manic symptoms worse. But when not acutely ill, the vast majority of bipolar patients do not experience psychotic symptoms; rather, their problems have to do with affect modulation and prevention of future breakdowns. For these people, the integrative model needs to be modified.

As compared with integrative groups for psychotic patients, non-psychosis bipolar groups commonly include a few formal presentations early in the life of the group on the illness (i.e., bipolar disorder) and its course, and on the characteristics of mood stabilizing medications and the need to be compliant with prescribed regimens. Later sessions are more unstructured and discussion-oriented. They deal with recognizing prodromal symptoms and ways of coping with them before they evolve into an acute manic or depressive episode; challenging distorted cognitions accompanying elevated and depressed emotional states; discussing important long-term psychodynamic issues associated with bipolar disorders; and learning ways of relating better with others, often via the here-and-now member interactions of the sessions. Like their psychosis counterpart, integrative bipolar groups have received empirical support to go along with clinical experience as to their characteristics and effectiveness.

To conclude, the integrative group therapy approach described in this book has been found to be a useful and successful adjunct to medications in helping patients who are suffering from schizophrenia spectrum and bipolar disorders. The use of this treatment model in both inpatient and outpatient settings should be incorporated into the overall treatment plan for people struggling with these serious mental conditions.

Index

A-B-C cognitive model 38–39, 42, 47, 84–85, 86, 99, 101, 126, 139, 141, 160, 175
Acceptance and Commitment Therapy (ACT) 48–49
Angst 21
anosognosia 17
Anxiety: effects on psychosis 21, 22, 25, 33, 44, 72, 77, 78, 127; in integrative non-psychosis bipolar groups 147, 153, 164, 168; in integrative psychosis groups 81, 87, 88, 94, 103, 104, 108, 111, 115, 116, 132, 133, 134, 176;
attachment theory 24–26, 103, 104

basic assumptions *see* Bion, W.
Beck, A.T. 37
Bellak, L. *see* ego functions
Bion, W. 28–29, 32
bipolar disorder: and maladaptive personality traits 158, 160, 161, 162, 163, 165, 169; combined treatment 157–158; didactic approaches: group therapy 152–153, group therapy research 153–156, theory 151; euthymic state 13, 145, 146, 159, 164, 165; group therapy and acute mania 146, 164–165, 177; nature of the disorder 145–147; non-didactic approaches: group therapy 149, group therapy research 149–151, theory 147–148; *see also* integrative group model for non-psychotic bipolar patients (clinical); integrative group model for non-psychotic bipolar patients (research); medications, use and compliance
Bleuler, E. 14

"booster" sessions 69, 152
Brooklyn State Hospital 27
Burlingame, G. 70, 72, 77

closed groups 95–96, 99
cognitive-behavioral group therapy *see* group therapy
cognitive-behavioral therapy (CBT) and psychosis: individual versus group 44–45; general treatment approach 38, 41–44; "second wave" 37; theory 40–41; "third wave" 47–51; *see also* group therapy for psychosis
cognitive remediation (CR) 43, 44, 70
combined therapy 114
Compassionate Mind Training 49
conjoint therapy 114

delusions *see* psychosis; *see* integrative group model (clinical)
Diagnostic and Statistical Manual of Mental Disorders, Fifth Edition (DSM-5): criteria for the psychoses 4–13
didactic approaches (cognitive-behavioral and psychoeducational): versus non-didactic approaches, rationale 60–61; *see also* bipolar disorder; *see also* group therapy: cognitive-behavioral (CBT); group therapy: psychoeducational; group therapy research
DSM-5 *see Diagnostic and Statistical Manual of Mental Disorders, Fifth Edition*

ego dystonic 23–24
ego functions 21–23, 39, 47, 78, 81, 175

ego syntonic 23
external stimulation-symptom
    relationship "U" curve *see* "U"
    curve external stimulation-symptom
    relationship

Francis, R. 4–9. 17–18, 78–79. 118–121
Frank, J.D. 33
Foulkes, S.H. 27–29, 32, 65

go-around 32, 35, 52, 80, 89, 90, 96, 97,
    98, 102
group analysis *see* Foulkes, S.H.
group-as-a-whole 28, 32, 36, 47, 90, 109
Group Climate Questionnaire, short-
    form (GCQ-S) 64–65, 131–134, 138,
    167–168; *see also* integrative group
    model (research); integrative group
    model for non-psychotic bipolar
    patients (research)
group cohesiveness 33, 34, 93; in
    integrative non-psychosis bipolar
    groups 164, 168; in integrative
    psychosis groups 132, 133, 134, 138,
    142
group dynamics and group stages
    29–30, 36, 64–65, 134, 165
group therapy for psychosis: cognitive-
    behavioral (CBT) 44–47, 174;
    combined treatment approaches
    51–53; group psychotherapy vs. group
    therapy 32–33; interpersonal 33–37,
    174; metaphors and 32, 79, 80, 81, 86;
    multi-family 20, 66, 71, 77; process-
    oriented 36–37; psychoanalytic/
    psychodynamic 26–32, 174;
    psychoeducational 18–20, 174; "third
    wave" 47–51; *see also* integrative group
    model (clinical, research); integrative
    group model for non-psychotic
    bipolar patients (clinical, research);
    Yalom, I.: inpatient groups
group therapy research: didactic 66–71;
    lessons learned 71–73; non-didactic
    61–66; *see also* integrative group
    model (research); integrative group
    model for non-psychotic bipolar
    patients (research)

hallucinations *see* psychosis; *see*
    integrative group model (clinical)
here-and-now 28, 31, 32–33, 35, 36; in
    integrative (psychosis) groups 78,
82, 83, 86, 88, 92, 101, 102, 103–104,
    108, 109, 115, 174, 175; in integrative
    non-psychosis bipolar groups 150,
    158, 160, 163, 164
heterogeneous groups 31, 34, 46, 52,
    70, 93–94
Hill Interaction Matrix (HIM-G)
    128–131, 139; *see also* integrative
    group model (research)
homogeneous groups 19, 34, 93–94,
    123
hypnagogic hallucinations 6, 42, 115
hypnopompic hallucinations 6, 42, 115

insight 16–18
Integrated Psychological Therapy
    (ITP) 66
integrative, use of term 77
integrative group model (clinical):
    advantages over non-integrative
    approaches 73,77–78, 174–175;
    anger in 94, 103, 105, 108–109,
    132, 134; background history
    76–77; clinical illustration of a
    typical session 90–92; cognitive-
    behavioral therapy (CBT) issues
    84–86; concurrent with individual
    therapy 114; confrontation 109;
    coping strategies 78–79, 84, 85, 86,
    88, 89–90, 92, 93–94, 105–107; cost-
    effectiveness 124–125, 135, 176–177;
    cotherapy 109–111; cultural issues
    122–124, 132–133, 142; definition
    77, 175; difficult patients 115–119;
    discussion topics in different
    settings 102–105; disruptive
    patients 115–116, eye contact in
    82, 83, 88; formal group exercises
    (discharged patient) 97–98; formal
    group exercises (new patient) 96–97,
    175–176; formal group exercises
    (therapist change) 98–99; group
    format in different settings 94–96;
    group goals 88–89, 98, 175–176;
    group goals, adjusting in different
    settings 98–102; group stages 134;
    homogeneous vs. heterogeneous
    groups 93–94; interpersonal issues
    82–83; medications 3,88, 104,
    105–106, 111–112, 119, 175, 176;
    monopolizing patients 116; overview
    78–88, 175–177; patient inclusion/
    exclusion 92–93, 177; patients

requesting frequent bathroom breaks 116; philosophy and religion 82, 120–121; pre-group intake 96–97; psychodynamic issues 79–81; psychoeducational issues 86–88; repeaters group 131, 138–139, 142, 176; safety 77, 88, 105, 132, 141; session sequence of events 89–90, 175; suicidal/homicidal patients 117; telepsychiatry 114, 125–126; therapist disclosure 114–115; therapist stance 107–109; training and supervision 121–122, 176; *see also* long-/short-term integrative groups

integrative group model (research): inpatient studies 127–133; lessons learned 141–142; outcome 141–142, 176; outpatient studies 133–141; process 142, 176; therapeutic factors 128, 130, 135, 136, 140, 141, 142, 176

integrative group model for non-psychotic bipolar patients (clinical): clinical illustration of atypical session 161–162; definition 158, 175; differences from integrative psychosis groups 163–164, 177; discussion topics 160–161; group format 165; group goals 158–160, 177; group process 165–167; medications 3, 146–147, 155–156, 159, 160, 161–162, 163, 169, 177; patient inclusion/exclusion 146–147, 164; suicidality 166; therapeutic factors 166–167; therapist stance 167

integrative group model for non-psychotic bipolar patients (research) 167–170

Integrative Group Outcome and Process Questionnaire 128–130, 135–136, 139–141; *see also* integrative group model (research)

Interactional Behavioral Training (IBT) 52

International Classification of Diseases, 10ᵗʰ Ed., Classification of Mental and Behavioural Disorders (ICD-10); criteria for the psychoses 13–14

Interpersonal and Social Rhythm Therapy (IPSRT) 157–158

interpersonal group therapy *see* group therapy

Interpersonal Therapy (IPT) 35–36

Kanas, N. air force study 76–77; integrative group studies (inpatient) 127–133; integrative group studies (outpatient) 133–141; integrative non-psychosis bipolar group studies 167–170; review of controlled group studies 61–63; *see also* integrative group model (clinical); integrative group model (research); integrative group model for non-psychotic bipolar patients (clinical); integrative group model for non-psychotic bipolar patients (research)

Klapman, J.W. 19, 32, 51–52

Lazell, E.W. 18–19, 32, 51, 174

Leszcz, M. *see* Yalom, I.

long-term integrative groups 80, 89, 98, 99, 101–102, 103, 104–105, 133–134, 139–141, 142, 163, 164, 176

loose associations *see* psychosis; *see* integrative group model (clinical)

Marmarosh, C.L. 24, 25, 26

Marsh, L.C. 19, 32

medications, use and compliance 3; in mood disorders 146–147, 155–156, 159, 160, 161–162, 163, 169, 177; in thought disorders 88, 104, 105–106, 111–112, 119, 175, 176

meditation 44, 47, 88, 119, 159–160

metacognitive approaches 47, 49–51, 71

Metacognitive Therapy (MCT) 49–51

metaphors 32, 79, 80, 81, 86

Method of Levels (MOL) 49

mindfulness-based approaches 47–48

mood disorders 1–2, 3, 9, 12–13, 52, 65–66, 145–146, 165; *see also* bipolar disorder; medications, use and compliance

Narrative Enhancement and Cognitive Therapy 46

negative symptoms 2, 3, 4, 8, 9, 11, 45–46, 118–119, 175; and homework 118

non-didactic approaches (interpersonal and psychoanalytic/psychodynamic): versus didactic approaches, rationale 60–61; *see also* bipolar disorder; group therapy: interpersonal; group therapy: psychoanalytic/psychodynamic; group therapy research non-integrative approaches, clinical limitations 77–78, 174–175

On Conquering Schizophrenia: From the Desk of a Therapist and Survivor, with Purview on Metaphysics, Philosophy, and Theology see Francis, R.
open groups 95, 99–101, 165

paranoia/paranoid 7, 25, 108, 118
Person-Based Cognitive Therapy (PBCT) 48
positive symptoms 2, 8, 25, 43, 50, 51, 68, 119
process-oriented group therapy *see* group therapy for psychosis: process oriented
Process-Oriented Psychoeducational (POP) group approach 52–53, 157
psychoanalytic/psychodynamic group therapy *see* group therapy
psychoanalytic theory of psychosis *see* psychosis: psychoanalytic theory of
psychodynamic groups 30–31, 60–61, 72
psychoeducational group therapy *see* group therapy
psychosis: dreams and 31; DSM-5 criteria 4–13; etiology and psychopathology 1–3, 45–46; psychoanalytic theory of 20–26; symptoms and signs, 4–9, 11; treatment (non-group) 3–4
psychotic-like conditions 13

reality sense 1, 13, 23–24, 39, 42, 47, 79, 81, 103, 175
reality testing 1, 13. 23–24, 39, 40, 41, 42, 45, 47, 81, 84, 101, 107, 122, 132
relaxation techniques 44, 88, 152, 159–160; *see also* meditation

Schilder, P. 26
schizophrenia spectrum 3, 10, 12
Schneider, K. 14, 103
self-stigma 20, 46, 98, 103, 104
Semrad, E.V. 26
short-term time-limited integrative groups 90, 93, 96, 99, 101, 103, 124, 130, 134–139, 140, 141, 142, 176, 177
slow-open groups 96, 99
social microcosm 36; *see also* here-and-now
social skills training (SST) 66, 67, 70, 71, 77
Stone, W.N. 3, 31–32, 33, 80, 81
stress-vulnerability model *see* vulnerability-stress model
Sullivan, H.S. 21

telepsychiatry and integrative groups 114, 125–126
there-and-then 31, 32, 104, 108, 109
"third wave" 47–51
thought disorders 3, 9, 10–12, 14, 60; *see also* medications, use and compliance

"U" curve external stimulation-symptom relationship 87, 105, 126, 139, 141, 158, 175

video games, as coping mechanism 106, 107
vulnerability-stress model 40, 42, 43, 47, 85–86, 99, 101, 105, 106, 126, 139, 141, 158, 175

Yalom, I.: bipolar groups 34, 147, 153, 168; inpatient groups 34–35, 37, 52, 94, 125; opinion of CBT groups 44; outpatient groups 26, 33–34, 36, 146, 150; therapeutic factors 34, 128, 166–167, 168